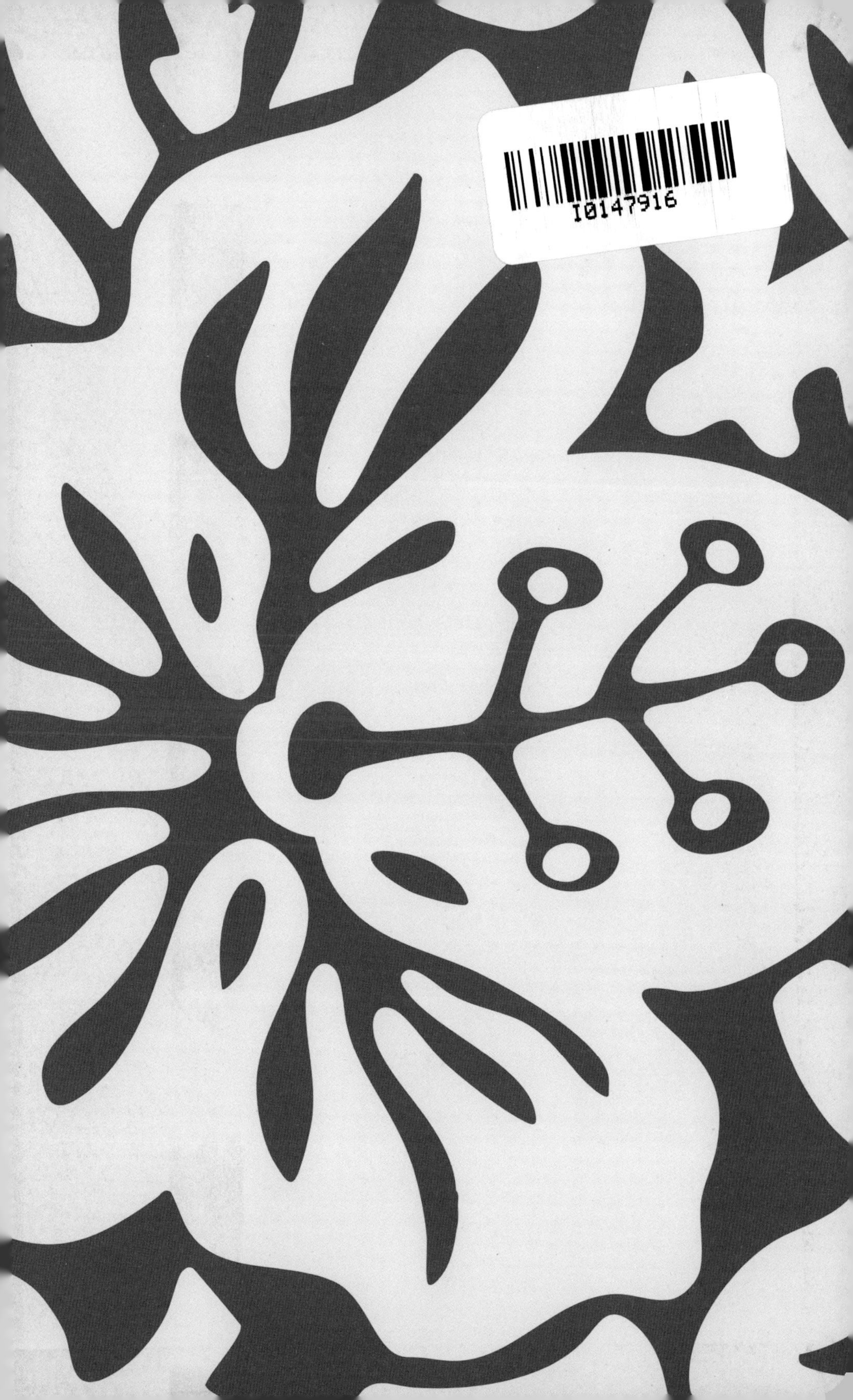
I0147916

Mayo Clinic

PREGNANCY JOURNAL

Weekly Reflections, Milestones and Expert Guidance

MAYO CLINIC

The publisher wishes to thank Marie E. Harke, R.N.

Image Credits All photographs and illustrations are copyright of Mayo Foundation for Medical Education and Research (MFMER) except for the following:
Cover: Alexander Ryabintsev/iStock/Getty Images, CSA Images/CSA Images/Getty Images
Interior: p. i, 13, 47, 94, 96, 97, 120, 125, 142 (bread, peach), 143 (milk, turkey), CREDIT: Alexander Ryabintsev/iStock/Getty Images; p. v, 14, 26, 38, 52, 62, 78, 90, 104, 122, 134, CREDIT: CSA Images/CSA Images/Getty Images; p. 3, CREDIT: Julia Ustugova/iStock/Getty Images; p. 9, 74, CREDIT: Naqiewei/DigitalVision Vectors/Getty Images; p. 16, CREDIT: timonko/iStock/Getty Images; p. 19, 140, CREDIT: MegaShabanov/iStock/Getty Images; p. 22, 113, CREDIT: Ivanova Nataliia/iStock/Getty Images; p. 31, CREDIT: Titrit/iStock/Getty Images Plus; p. 44, 83, 88, 137, CREDIT: Olga Shevchenko/iStock/Getty Images; p. 51, CREDIT: Thirteen-Fifty/iStock/Getty Images; p. 61, 98, CREDIT: Danang Setyo Nugroho/iStock/Getty Images; p. 67, CREDIT: budi priyanto/iStock/Getty Images; p. 99, CREDIT: Olga Ubirailo/iStock/Getty Images; p. 119, CREDIT: Tetiana Garkusha/iStock/Getty Images; p. 141, CREDIT: Toltemara/iStock/Getty Images; p. 142 (pepper), CREDIT: Olha Furmaniuk/iStock/Getty Images

MAYO CLINIC PRESS
200 First St. SW
Rochester, MN 55905
MCPress.MayoClinic.org

ISBN 979-8-88770-401-2

Library of Congress Control Number: 2025032243

Library of Congress Cataloging-in-Publication Data is available upon request.

Printed in China
First printing: 2026

Contents

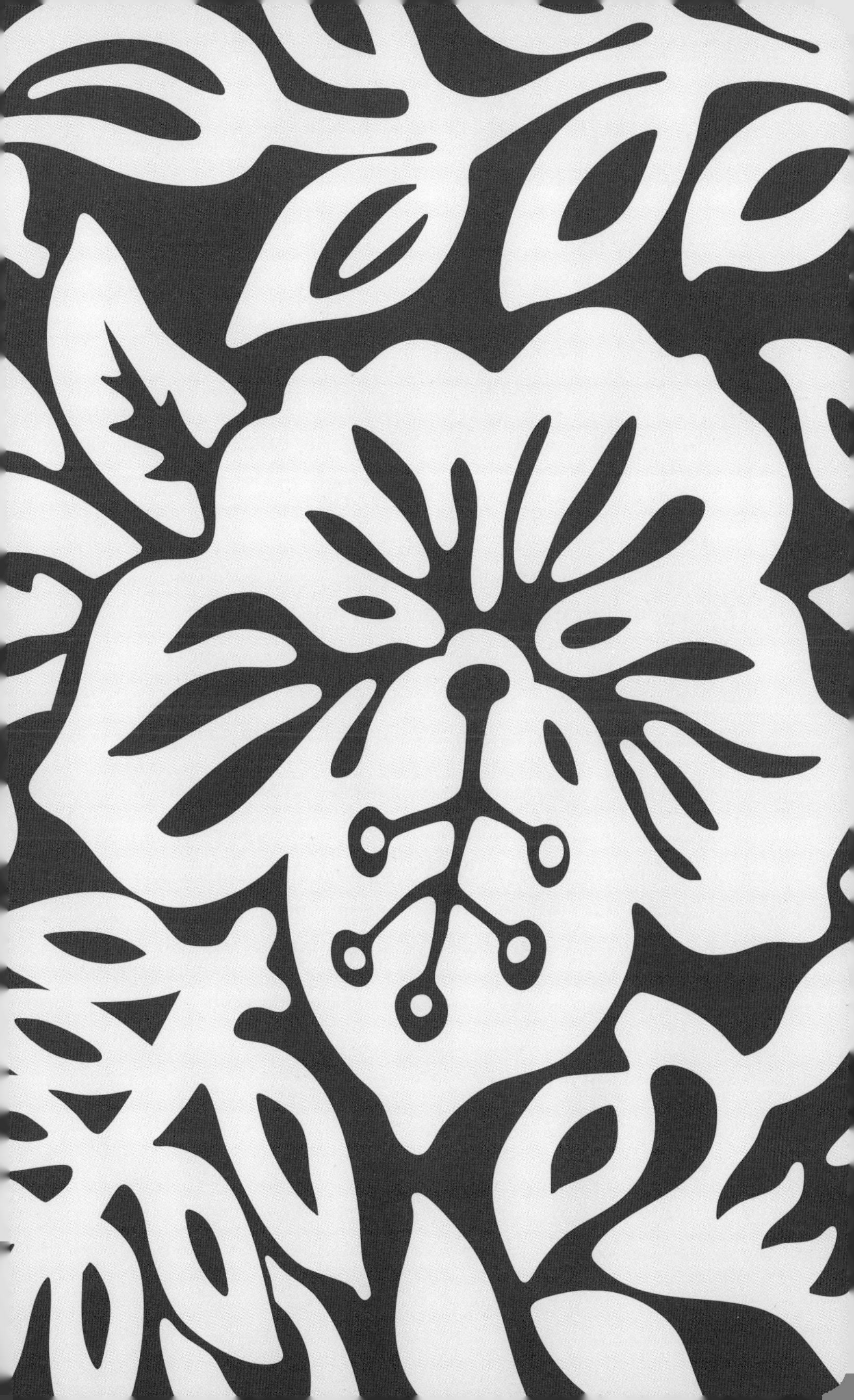

Introduction

Congratulations! If you've picked up this journal, you've likely begun a great adventure. Pregnancy can be an exciting time. It can also be highly emotional, full of both joy and worry. This journal is designed to help you mark this major moment in your life, record key information and organize your thoughts as you prepare for the birth of your child.

For many, pregnancy is a time of looking to the future. This journal helps you consider practical questions in planning for your labor and raising your child. But pregnancy is a time for looking inward and stopping to consider the present, too. This journal invites you to pause and reflect on pregnancy milestones, from first ultrasounds to packing your hospital bag. It provides a space for you to note symptoms and changes in your rapidly changing body. It encourages you to explore your thoughts on everything from baby gear to parenting styles.

The prompts here echo the book *Mayo Clinic Guide to a Healthy Pregnancy*, a comprehensive guide that includes week-by-week developments for you and baby. Though the book and journal don't need to be used together, they make great companions. Each page of this journal offers insights and key medical information to help empower you in caring for yourself and your baby. And the book makes a great go-to reference for all of your pregnancy questions.

Why 10 months? And where's month 1?

Wait — pregnancy lasts nine months, right? So why do we list 10 months? In determining your due date and monitoring your progress, your healthcare team works from a 40-week calendar. If you think of a month as four weeks, take 40 divided by 4, and that equals 10 months. However, most calendar months are a little more than four weeks, and those extra days add up. So a typical pregnancy is closer to nine calendar months. Because your healthcare team will track your pregnancy by week, we've opted to list 10 four-week months.

You'll notice that the first month of pregnancy is absent from this journal. That's because people don't typically know they're pregnant until the end of month 1. This journal begins weekly topics with month 2. But first, if you've recently found out you're expecting, turn to "Beginning your journey," a collection of prompts for people who are beginning to take stock of all that their pregnancy entails.

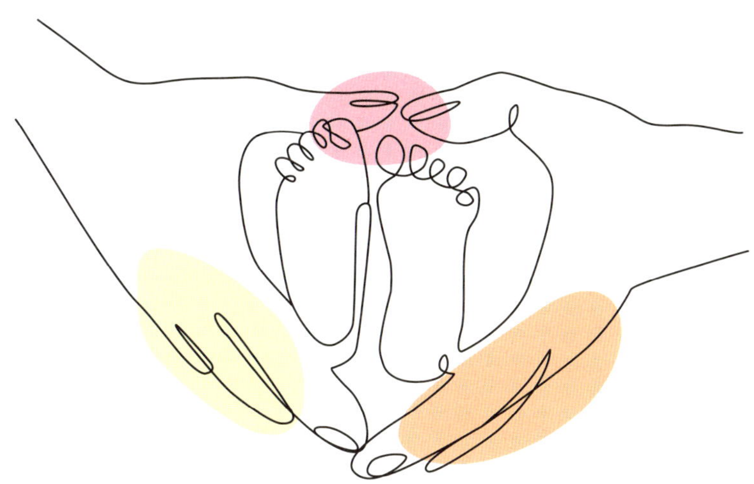

Beginning your journey

You're pregnant!

The journey to pregnancy can be straightforward or very complex. No matter how the pregnancy comes to be, it can be an emotional roller coaster. Take some time to reflect on the path to this pregnancy. How long was your journey to conception? What emotions did you feel as you tried to get pregnant? Did you experience any struggles along the way? When and how did you find out you're pregnant? What was it like to learn about this pregnancy?

First trimester to-do list:

Stay on top of things during your pregnancy with checklists for each trimester! Here are some things to consider during your first trimester. Continue reading to explore some of these items in more detail. And if you want, fill in the blank spaces with any additional items you want to consider.

Want to keep this checklist on hand for easy reference? Scan the QR code on the last page of the book to find a downloadable version of the checklist for each trimester.

- [ ] Contact your insurance to check on what coverage and costs to expect for prenatal and childbirth care
- [ ] Find a prenatal healthcare professional
- [ ] Schedule and have your first prenatal visit
- [ ] Schedule follow-up prenatal visits
- [ ] Decide on an exercise plan
- [ ] Consider any diet changes to support your nutritional needs in pregnancy (see page 142)
- [ ] Take stock of your daily caffeine, sleep, medications and other lifestyle factors, and consider changes needed
- [ ] Consider your financial plans with a partner, support person or on your own
- [ ] Discuss prenatal testing with your partner or support person and your healthcare team
- [ ] Have your first ultrasound
- [ ] ______
- [ ] ______

Choosing a healthcare professional

Finding the right healthcare professional to help you prepare for childbirth can make a big difference in your experience. Plenty of options are available for prenatal care, birth locations and birth preferences.

- Obstetrician-gynecologists, also called OB-GYNs, specialize in women's health and can handle most problems that arise during pregnancy.
- Midwives provide pre-conception, maternity and postpartum care for low-risk pregnancies.
- Family physicians care for the whole family through all stages of life. However, some may not handle pregnancies.
- Maternal-fetal medicine specialists, also known as perinatologists, specialize in high-risk pregnancies.

To help you decide, here are some suggestions and things to consider:

- See what options your insurance company covers.
- Consult your regular healthcare team, clinic or hospital for who provides care and recommendations.
- Check that the professional you want is qualified, can answer questions between appointments, is compatible with your personality and is able to fulfill your wants and needs.

What are your personal preferences for a healthcare professional, and why? Are your options limited now, or might they possibly be limited in the future, by factors you can't control? What qualities should your healthcare team have to help you trust them, especially during the crucial moments of labor and birth?

Advocating for yourself

A trusted healthcare professional is a key partner in your pregnancy. But you are also an essential partner in your care. Throughout your pregnancy, and afterward, it's smart to be aware of what's happening in your body and the options available to you at each step. Engaging in your healthcare decisions empowers you to be your own advocate — to use your voice and speak up for your needs.

Do you feel comfortable voicing your needs? What fears or concerns do you have around advocating for yourself? What are some ways you can empower yourself to be a partner in your own care during this pregnancy and beyond?

Inequity in pregnancy health

Racial and ethnic minorities are more likely to face issues such as preterm birth, gestational diabetes, injury during childbirth and life-threatening complications during pregnancy. If you are part of a minority population, find a professional who understands healthcare inequity and can provide you with more personalized care. And if you initially chose a professional that doesn't meet your needs, it's OK to find someone different. Recommendations from friends, family and online reviews are good places to start.

New and mixed feelings

Whether your pregnancy was planned or unplanned, you may have conflicting feelings about it. Even if you're thrilled about being pregnant, you may worry about your baby or the changes that come with pregnancy and parenthood. These concerns are natural and normal. What emotions about your pregnancy have you experienced? What worries do you have?

Did you know?

Within 4 to 5 days after fertilization, your developing baby (now made up of about 500 cells) reaches the inside of your uterus.

Circle any emotions that describe how you're feeling now. You can also write in other emotions you feel if they aren't listed.

Happy

Confused

Excited

Hopeful

Surprised

Worried

Anxious

Fearful

Stressed

Confident

Overwhelmed

Mood swings

As you adjust to being pregnant, you may experience a wide range of emotions and changing emotions from day to day or even over the course of a single day. It may feel like you're on an emotional roller coaster. Have you noticed any mood swings yet? How could your partner, family or other support system help when you experience this common pregnancy symptom?

Did you know?

By the end of your pregnancy, your blood volume will have increased 30% to 50%.

Healthy choices during pregnancy

A new baby on the way is a great reason to take stock of your current lifestyle. Pregnancy provides many people with the motivation to eat well, exercise more and minimize risky habits.

Think about your current diet, exercise and other lifestyle habits. What changes would you like to make, if any? Do you feel confident about making any changes you're planning, or do you have any concerns? How do you envision these changes affecting your life beyond your pregnancy? Discuss your plans, as well as any medications you're taking, with your healthcare team.

Things to consider for a healthy pregnancy

- *Nutrition:* Eat a variety of nutritious foods and take a prenatal vitamin with sufficient folic acid. Turn to page 142 for more guidance on what to eat for the energy and nutrients you need in pregnancy.
- *Caffeine:* Research is ongoing, but less than 200mg per day is generally thought to be safe.
- *Activity:* Move your body every day. This can be as simple as taking a walk! If you already exercise, don't presume you have to change much, but talk with your healthcare team.

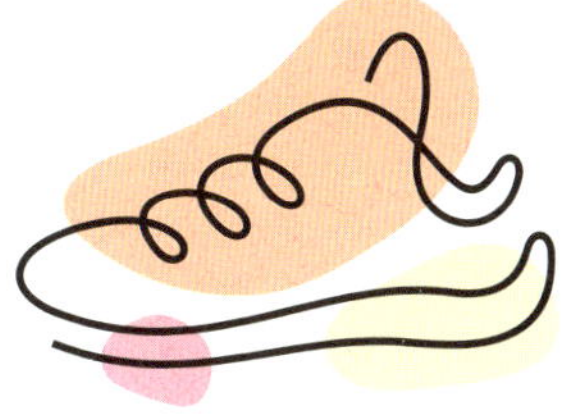

- *Harmful substances:* Avoid alcohol, marijuana, cigarettes and vaping.
- *Medication use:* Avoid certain over-the-counter medications, including common cold medications. Check the table on page 145 for guidance. Talk with your healthcare team about any prescription medications you are taking.
- *Vaccines:* Talk with your healthcare team about vaccines recommended in pregnancy to help protect you and baby.

You can find more answers to common questions about having a healthy pregnancy in ***Mayo Clinic Guide to a Healthy Pregnancy***.

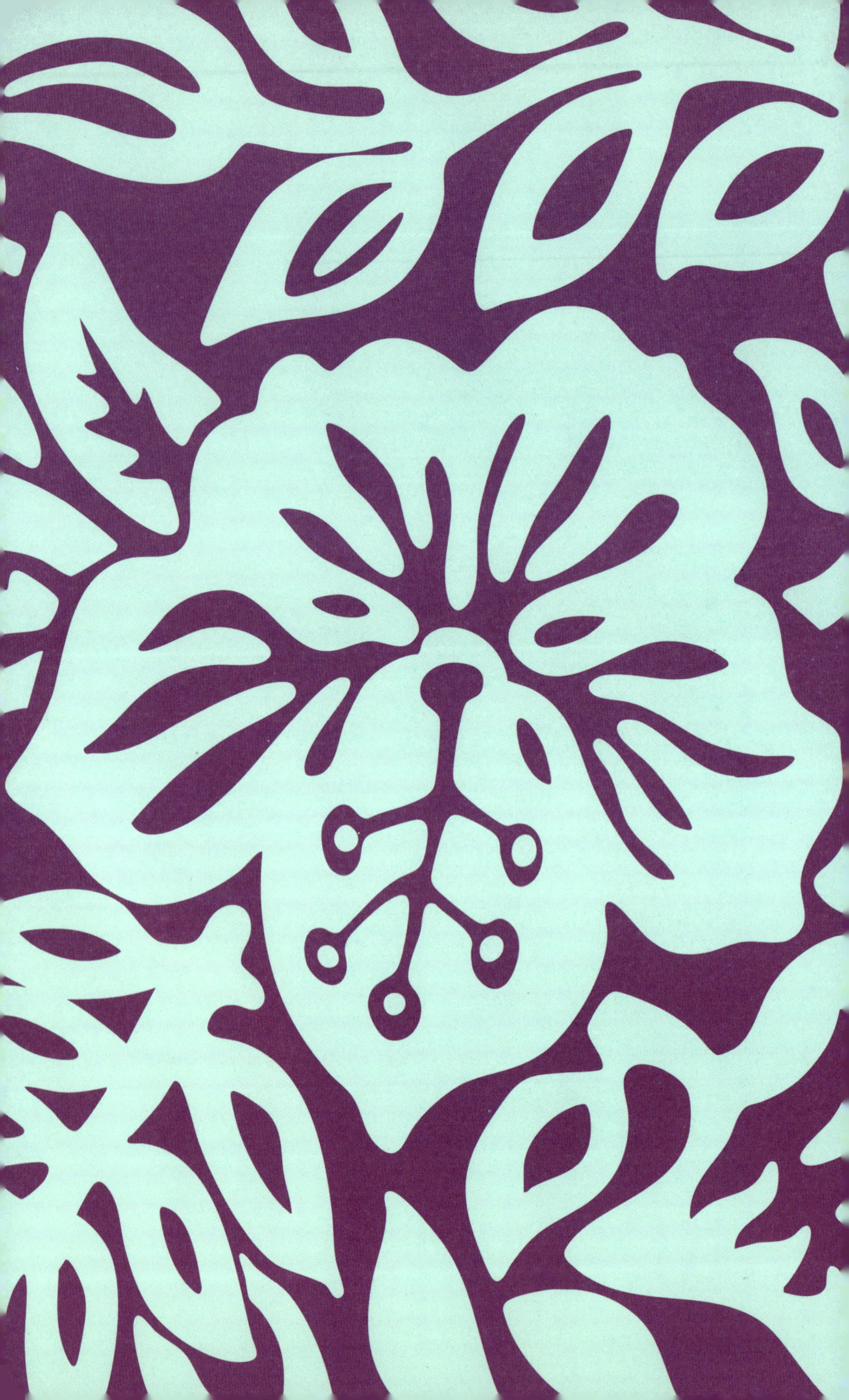

Month 2

Monthly check-in

Date: ______

Weeks of gestation: ______

Blood pressure: ______

Weight: ______

Baby's heart rate: ______

What was the most exciting thing that happened this last month?

What was the funniest moment?

Cravings, body changes, and other monthly notes:

What questions do you have for your healthcare professional?

Week 5

Your relationship with your partner

If you have a partner, it's important for you both to talk openly and honestly to manage stress in your relationship. For example, you may have reacted differently to learning you're pregnant. During pregnancy, there may be times when your interest in sexual activity doesn't match up, or you have different ideas for planning and parenting. All of these differences are opportunities to connect and discuss what you're thinking and feeling.

How do you think your relationship might be affected by your pregnancy? Are there certain ways you'd like to be supported, such as making healthy lifestyle changes or shifting household responsibilities? What specific steps can you and your partner take to openly communicate with each other?

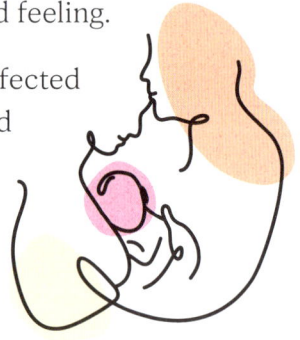

Did you know?

During pregnancy, your heart will grow to accommodate the increase in blood volume, heart rate and cardiac output.

Week
6

What kind of parent do you want to be?

Anticipation is a normal part of making the transition to parenthood. This includes thinking about what you'll be like as a parent. You probably have already been collecting ideas about how to be a good parent. And they are probably based on the parenting you received as a child and your observations of other families.

What stands out to you about how you were raised? What observations of other families have made an impression on you? With these influences, what is your vision for your own parenting style?

Sharing your worries and concerns

During your second month of pregnancy, the initial excitement about the baby may be mixed with anxiety. You may worry about your baby's health. You may also worry about other things, such as coping with pregnancy, changes at work, arranging for child care and more. What are some of the worries and concerns you have right now? Who can you share these worries and concerns with?

If troubling thoughts and feelings persist and you find them distressing, consider talking to a member of your healthcare team. They may refer you to a therapist or counselor, who can help you manage anxiety.

Week 7

Your body changes: Coping with morning sickness and other symptoms

The second month of pregnancy brings enormous changes for your body, and you're likely to start feeling it! Common discomforts and annoyances of early pregnancy include nausea and vomiting, heartburn, insomnia and feeling like you constantly need to pee. You may also notice an increased heart rate which can cause fatigue, dizziness and headaches. Your breasts may also start feeling fuller and heavier as well as tender, tingly or sore. Morning sickness — which may hit at any time of day — can be especially challenging to cope with in your daily routine.

What body changes have you experienced so far? What techniques have you found to relieve problematic symptoms? If you haven't experienced any body changes yet, how can you plan ahead to cope with them? Do you have any concerns to bring up with your healthcare team?

Did you know?

Your baby's first heartbeats occur at 21 to 22 days after conception. And by week 8, your baby's heart is pumping at about 150 beats a minute, about twice the adult rate.

Tips for dealing with nausea

- *Choose foods carefully:* Find foods that are bland or dry, easy to digest and lower in fat. This might sound boring, but it'll help you feel better!
- *Snack often:* This can be in the morning before getting out of bed or right after getting up, and throughout the day.
- *Drink fluids:* Sipping water and ginger ale may help, or try sucking on hard candy, ice chips or ice pops.
- *Pay attention to triggers:* Avoid foods or smells that might make your nausea worse.
- *Get fresh air:* Opening windows or going for a walk can help.
- *Take care with prenatal vitamins:* Try taking prenatal vitamins at night or with a snack.
- *Try acupressure and acupuncture:* Though not scientifically proven to be effective, some may find these therapies to be helpful.

Did you know?

If this is your first pregnancy, your uterus has previously been about the size of a pear. Now it's starting to expand. By the time you deliver your baby, it will have expanded in volume to about 500 times its original size.

Week 8

Preparing for your first prenatal checkup

Near the end of this month or in the following weeks, you'll see your pregnancy care team for your first prenatal visit. What questions do you have for your care team? Make sure to write them down ahead of time so you don't forget in the moment. What excites you about this first checkup? What fears do you have about it?

First appointment checklist

At your first prenatal appointment, you'll discuss your medical history. You will likely cover the following topics:

- [ ] Details of any previous pregnancies
- [ ] The typical length of time between your periods
- [ ] The first day of your last period
- [ ] Your use of contraceptives
- [ ] Prescription or over-the-counter medications you're taking
- [ ] Allergies you have
- [ ] Medical conditions or diseases you have had or now have
- [ ] Past surgeries, if any
- [ ] Your work environment
- [ ] Your lifestyle behaviors, such as exercise, diet, smoking or exposure to secondhand smoke and use of alcoholic beverages or recreational drugs
- [ ] Risk factors for sexually transmitted infections — such as you or your partner having more than one sexual partner
- [ ] Past or present medical problems, such as diabetes, high blood pressure (hypertension), lupus or depression in your or your partner's immediate family — parents and siblings
- [ ] Family histories, on both sides, of babies with congenital abnormalities or genetic diseases
- [ ] Details of your home environment, such as whether you feel safe and supported at home

Reflecting on your first prenatal checkup

The first prenatal checkup can be an exciting milestone. Use this space to reflect on your experience. How did the checkup go? What did you learn about your pregnancy and your baby? If you had an ultrasound, what was it like? What were the results?

Questions after your first prenatal checkup

What questions did the appointment inspire? Consider following up with your care team for any short-term questions. Also write down anything that you want to remember to ask at future prenatal appointments.

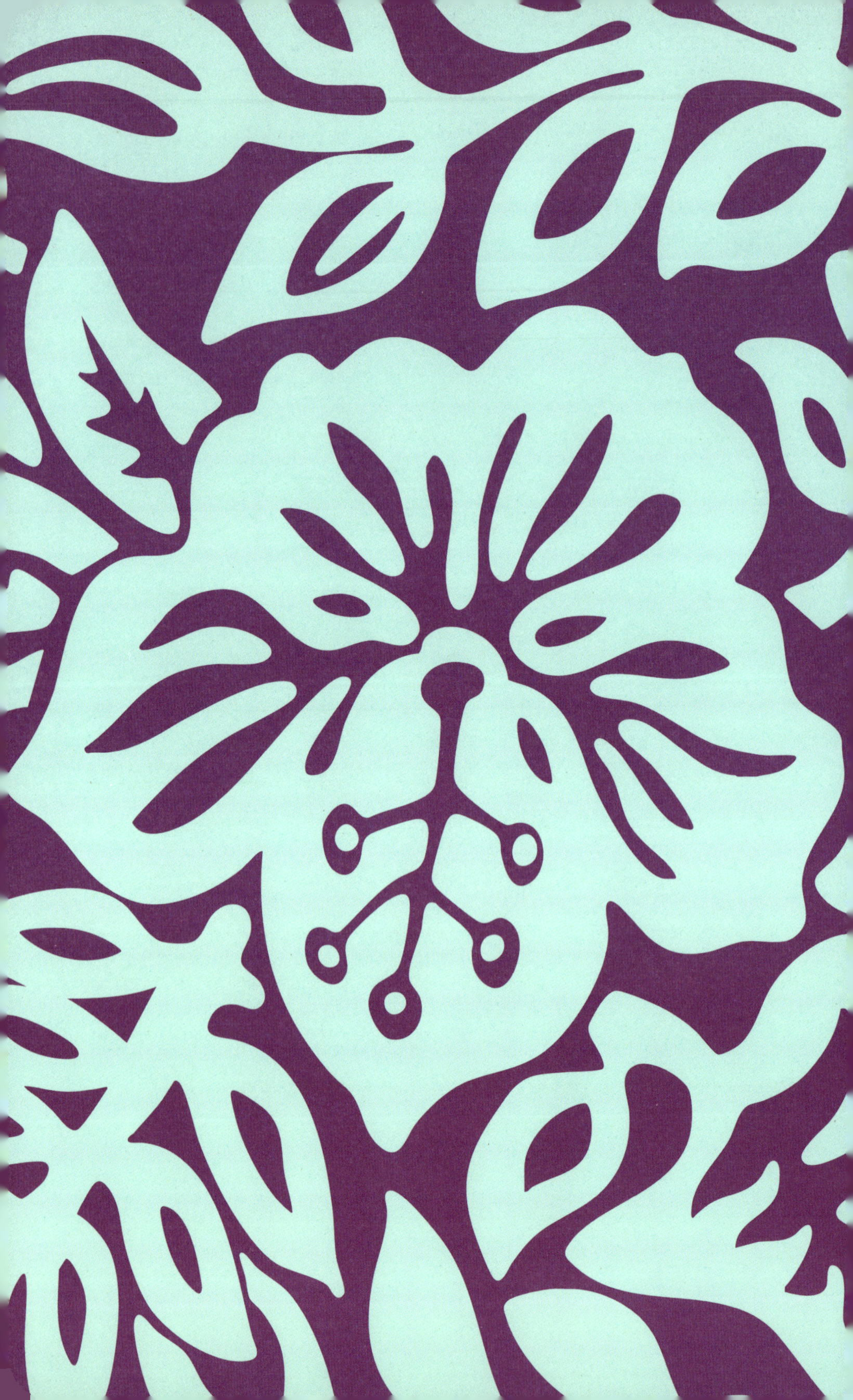

Month 3

Monthly check-in

Date: ____________________

Weeks of gestation: ____________________

Blood pressure: ____________________

Weight: ____________________

Baby's heart rate: ____________________

What was the most exciting thing that happened this last month?

What was the funniest moment?

Cravings, body changes, and other monthly notes:

What questions do you have for your healthcare professional?

Week 9

Good to know: Recognizing perinatal depression and anxiety

Depression and anxiety can occur during pregnancy. If low mood or worry lasts for longer than two weeks and interferes with your ability to eat, sleep, work, concentrate, relate to others or enjoy life, you may be experiencing depression or anxiety.

Symptoms of depression include loss of interest in normal daily activities; feeling sad, helpless or hopeless; fatigue; sleep disturbances; and impaired thinking or concentration. Symptoms of anxiety include persistent worrying; feeling nervous, restless or tense; having a sense of impending danger; and having trouble concentrating or sleeping.

Do you recognize any symptoms of depression or anxiety in yourself? What are your symptoms like? Do you have a history of depression or anxiety? If so, what treatments have been effective? Who can you talk to about any concerns you may have around treatment during pregnancy?

Reach out to your healthcare team right away if you believe you have depression or anxiety. They can help you get the treatment you need.

Depression and anxiety are serious concerns that require treatment. Ignoring them can put you and your baby at risk. Often, depression and anxiety that occur during pregnancy are treated with counseling and behavioral therapy. Antidepressant medications may be used as well. Many of these medications appear to carry little risk to developing babies, while untreated moderate to severe depression can pose multiple health risks for both the parent and baby.

Risks of stopping depression and anxiety treatment in pregnancy

For the pregnant person	For baby
Worsening symptoms	Inadequate growth during pregnancy
Poor self-care	Low birth weight
Inadequate weight gain or weight loss	Developmental delay after birth
Suicidal thoughts or behaviors	Cognitive impairment after birth
Preterm labor	
Difficulty bonding with newborn	
Inability to cope with stress of parenting	

Your body changes: Early pregnancy symptoms

Some of the discomforts and annoyances of early pregnancy, such as morning sickness, fatigue and feeling like you constantly need to pee, may be particularly troublesome this month. But usually, this is only temporary.

This month, you may also have insomnia and vivid dreams, slightly blurred vision, twinges, cramps or pulling in the lower abdomen and weight gain.

What new body changes have arisen over the last month? What strategies can you use to cope with problematic symptoms? Do you have any concerns to bring up with your healthcare team?

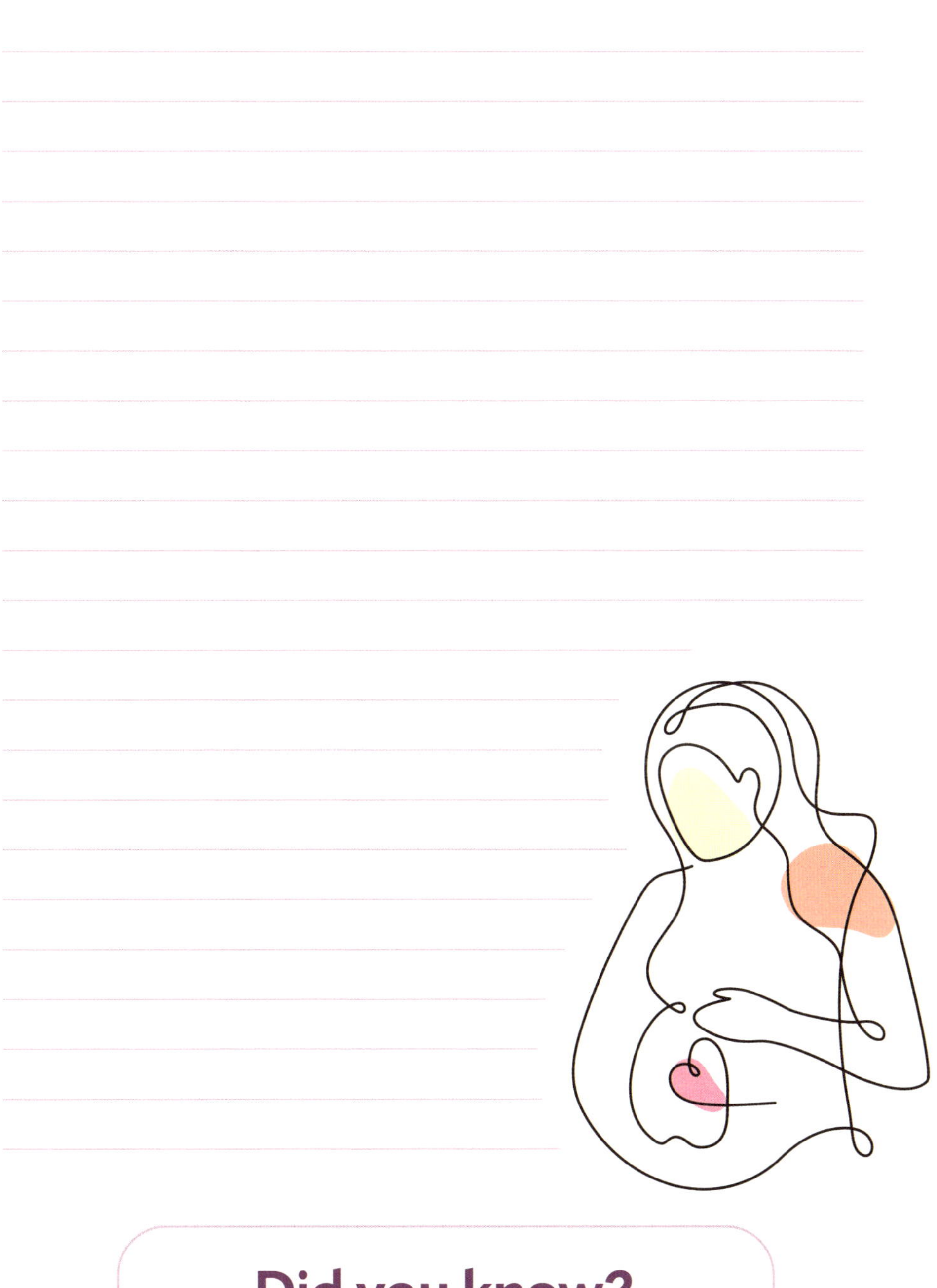

Did you know?

By week 10, all of your baby's vital organs have begun to form. And your baby is producing almost 250,000 new neurons every minute.

Your body changes: Your pelvic floor

Your pelvic floor muscles surround and support your bladder, vagina and rectum. They stabilize your pelvic bones, support your spine and help control the release of urine, stool and gas. During pregnancy, your pelvic floor muscles work harder to support the weight of your growing baby while being softened by your pregnancy hormones to prepare for labor. This can cause a feeling of pressure or heaviness. You might feel like you have to pee more often, and you might not be able to hold your pee like you used to. Talk to your care team if you are very uncomfortable when doing your daily activities. Pelvic floor physical therapy may help.

Other common symptoms you may want to talk with your provider about include:

- Constipation and straining with bowel movements
- Vaginal pain with intercourse that is not improved by changing positions or using lubricants
- Burning with urination
- Fever with urinary symptoms
- Seeing or feeling tissue bulging from the vagina
- Low back, pubic or hip pain

Whether or not you have symptoms related to your pelvic floor, now is a great time to start doing pelvic floor exercises if you haven't already. A strong pelvic floor can make pregnancy more comfortable and reduce your chances of having pelvic floor issues later on. For more information on pelvic floor exercises, see page 81.

Week
11

Prenatal testing

At this month's prenatal checkup, a member of your healthcare team may talk with you about prenatal testing for fetal abnormalities. Or this may have been discussed at your first prenatal appointment. Prenatal tests screen for certain problems with your baby's health, generally by way of a blood test or ultrasound exam. Some common conditions these tests may screen for are Down syndrome, neural tube defects, abdominal wall defects and chromosomal abnormalities and disorders. Some prenatal tests are optional, while others are highly recommended or required. You may want to check on which tests your insurance will cover, as coverage varies for tests that are considered optional.

What questions do you have about prenatal testing? What tests would you like to have done and why? How would you and your partner respond to abnormal results?

Boy or girl?

In the coming weeks, you may be able to find out the sex of your little one — if you want to. Certain prenatal tests give parents the option to learn their baby's sex as part of the results. Otherwise, many parents find out the big news of baby's sex from a standard ultrasound done around 18 to 20 weeks.

Do you want to know your baby's sex before the birth? Does your partner agree with you? If you want to know, how will you use this information as you prepare for your baby's arrival?

Week

12

12-week ultrasound

You may have had an ultrasound at your 12-week prenatal appointment. If you did, how did it go? What were the results?

If you'd like, tape or glue a copy of your ultrasound picture below. (The pocket inside the back cover can hold additional photos.) Add any notes you may want on memorable observations that were made and on any measurements taken during the ultrasound.

Prenatal test results

If you had any other prenatal testing done, what information did you learn about your baby? How do you feel about it?

Hopes for baby

As you reach the end of your first trimester, your baby may feel more real to you, which can be exciting. And, with the risk of miscarriage now greatly reduced, you may be thinking more about your wishes, how you will parent and more. What hopes do you have for your baby right now? How do you envision yourself raising this baby? What kind of relationship would you like to have with your baby? Consider writing this as a letter to your baby.

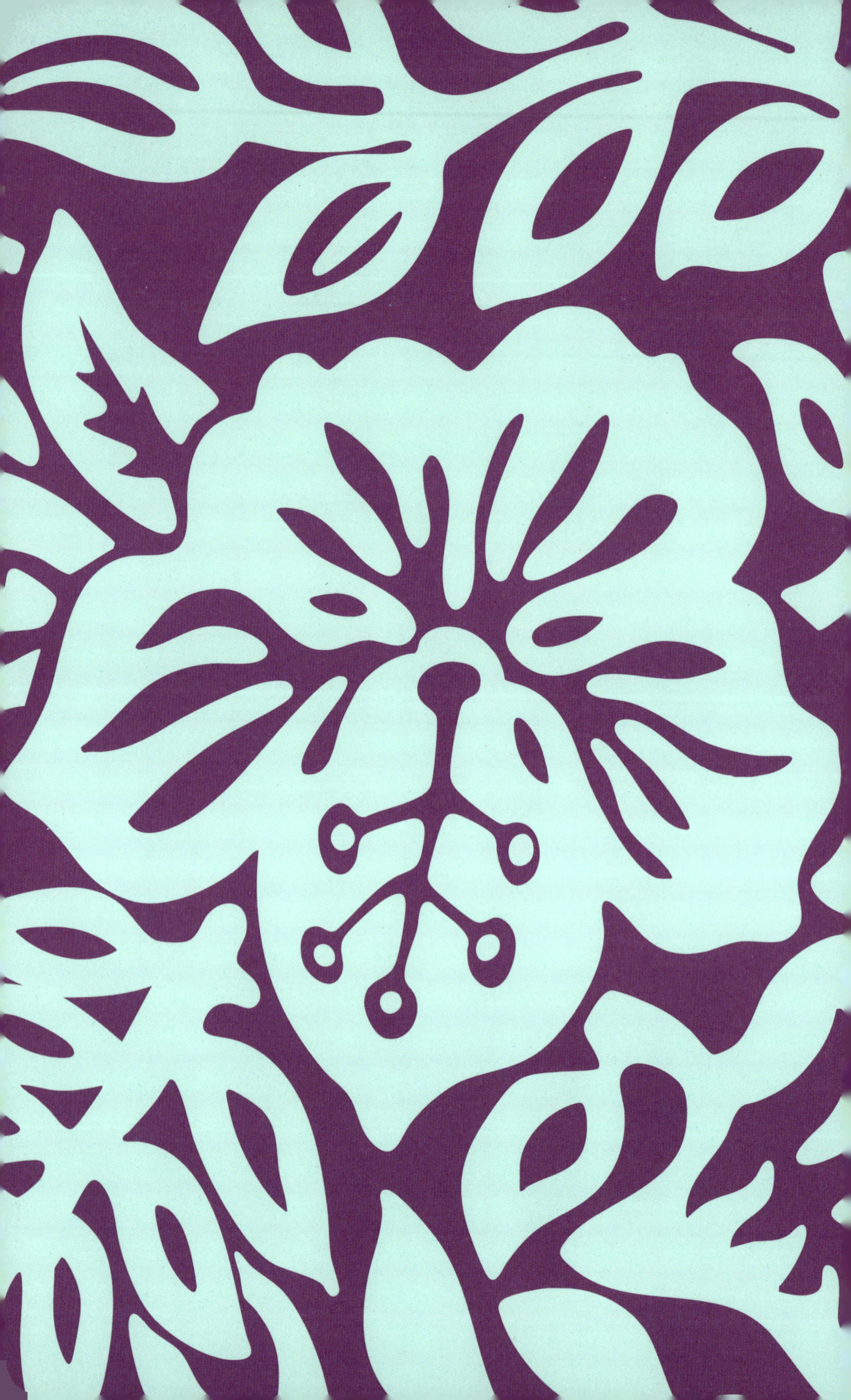

Month 4

Monthly check-in

Date: ____________________

Weeks of gestation: ____________________

Blood pressure: ____________________

Weight: ____________________

Baby's heart rate: ____________________

What was the most exciting thing that happened this last month?

What was the funniest moment?

Cravings, body changes, and other monthly notes:

What questions do you have for your healthcare professional?

Week

13

Your baby's growth: First trimester

As the first trimester ends, your baby has been transforming quickly! All of your baby's organs, nerves and muscles have taken basic form and are beginning to function together. Growth continues at a rapid pace, but your baby is still small — just 2 to 3 ounces as this month kicks off.

Your baby's eyes and ears are now clearly identifiable, although the eyelids are fused together to protect the developing eyes. Tissue that will become bone is developing around your baby's head and within the arms and legs. Your baby is now moving their body in a jerky fashion, flexing their arms and kicking their legs. Your baby may be able to reach a thumb to their mouth, and sucking may begin within a few weeks.

Is baby's development in line with what you expected by this time? Does learning about baby's growth make you relate differently to your baby or your body?

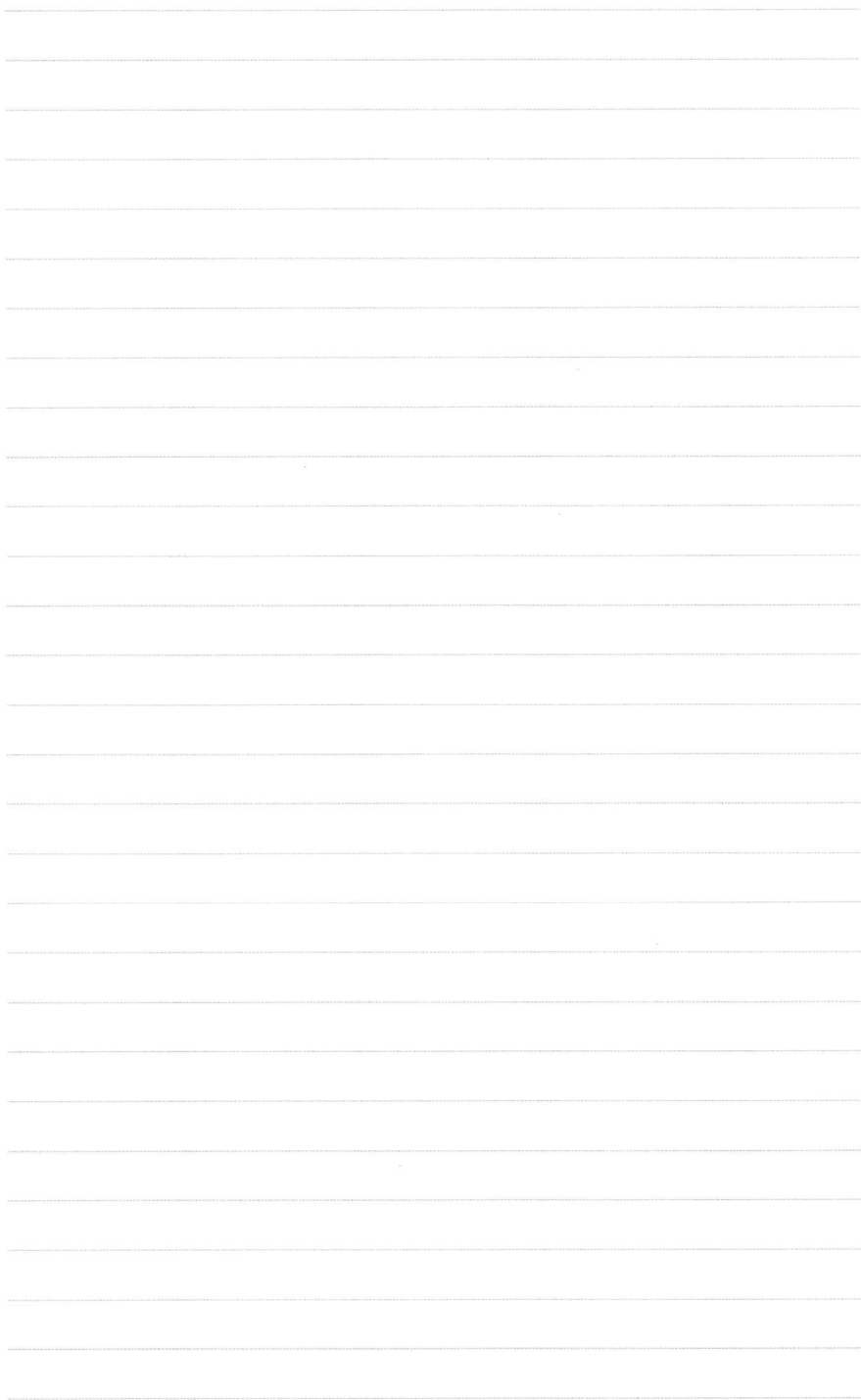

Week 14

When you're feeling productive

If your first-trimester pregnancy symptoms are easing, now is a great time for you and your partner to jump on some "housekeeping" tasks, such as planning for childbirth classes, checking parental leave policies and thinking about child care for when you go back to work. If you're not feeling up for these tasks, don't worry. There's still plenty of time.

What tasks do you have on your to-do list? If you're not sure what to add, use the sample list on the next page to get started. Do you feel up for doing any tasks in the coming weeks? Who can help you with these tasks?

Second trimester to-do list:

Here are some things to consider as you enter your second trimester. Continue reading to learn more about some of these tasks. You can also fill in the blank spaces with any additional items you want to consider.

- [ ] Consider if and how you want to share your news
- [ ] Schedule follow-up prenatal appointments
- [ ] Sign up for childbirth classes
- [ ] Get familiar with maternity and paternity leave policies
- [ ] Look into child care
- [ ] Find a healthcare professional for your baby
- [ ] Think about how you want to feed your baby
- [ ] Have your mid-pregnancy ultrasound
- [ ] Do your glucose test
- [ ] ______
- [ ] ______
- [ ] ______
- [ ] ______
- [ ] ______
- [ ] ______
- [ ] ______
- [ ] ______
- [ ] ______

Sharing your news!

You may have begun announcing your pregnancy more widely at this point in your pregnancy. Who did you tell first? What was it like to share the news with various people in your life? How did you tell them?

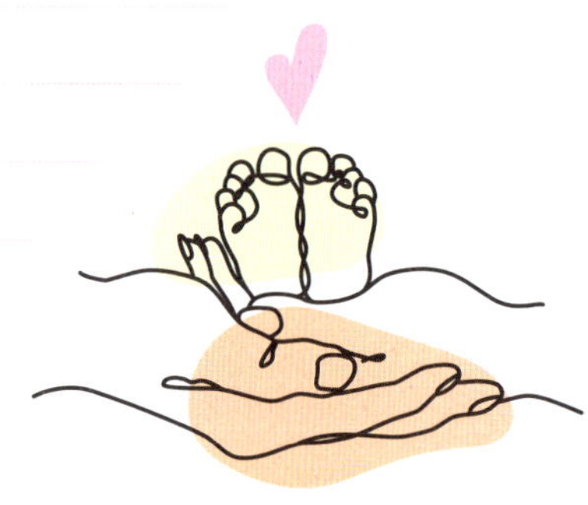

Nurturing your relationships

Pregnancy and preparing for a new baby can take time, energy and focus away from your other roles and relationships. How have your relationships with friends and family members been affected by this pregnancy? What changes would you like to see as the pregnancy continues? How can you communicate with your loved ones to determine how you can best support each other?

Week 15

Your body changes: The golden period of pregnancy

This month begins with what's sometimes called the golden period of pregnancy. The nausea and fatigue of early pregnancy have typically lessened, the discomforts of the third trimester haven't yet begun and your risk of miscarriage is now greatly reduced.

This month, certain areas of your skin and your areolas may darken in color. You may also have constipation, increased vaginal discharge, iron deficiency anemia, lower blood pressure, nasal congestion, nosebleeds and bleeding gums when you brush your teeth. As baby grows, you may also feel more aches and pains (including back pain), heartburn, a changing center of gravity, leg cramps and faster breathing.

What new body changes have you noticed over the last month? What strategies can you use to cope with problematic symptoms? Do you have any concerns to bring up with your healthcare team?

Body image

While some people love the physical changes of pregnancy, others struggle with them. Expressing your feelings, learning as much as you can about pregnancy and seeking mental health support can help you get comfortable with how your body is changing. Getting regular physical activity and trying prenatal yoga or massage if your care team says it's OK can also help you stay active and help you feel better.

How have the physical changes of pregnancy affected you so far? How are you feeling about your body changing as the pregnancy progresses? What techniques are you open to trying if you want to get more comfortable with your changing body?

Did you know?

Your baby's facial muscles are developing, and baby will soon be able to make a variety of expressions. Though these movements aren't conscious expressions of emotions, an ultrasound may catch baby squinting or frowning at you!

Week 16

Thinking ahead to child care

A common decision for many working parents is what they will do once the baby is born. Have you determined whether you and your partner will both return to work? How did you come to that decision? If you're undecided, how do your financial needs, your desire to maintain a career, your desire to be a full-time parent and your ability to manage stress affect your decision?

If you and your partner will both return to work or you're undecided, it's best to explore your options and secure child care as early as possible. What child care options have you considered? How do your budget, your expectations and your family dynamics affect your child care options? Who can help you make the best decision for you and your family?

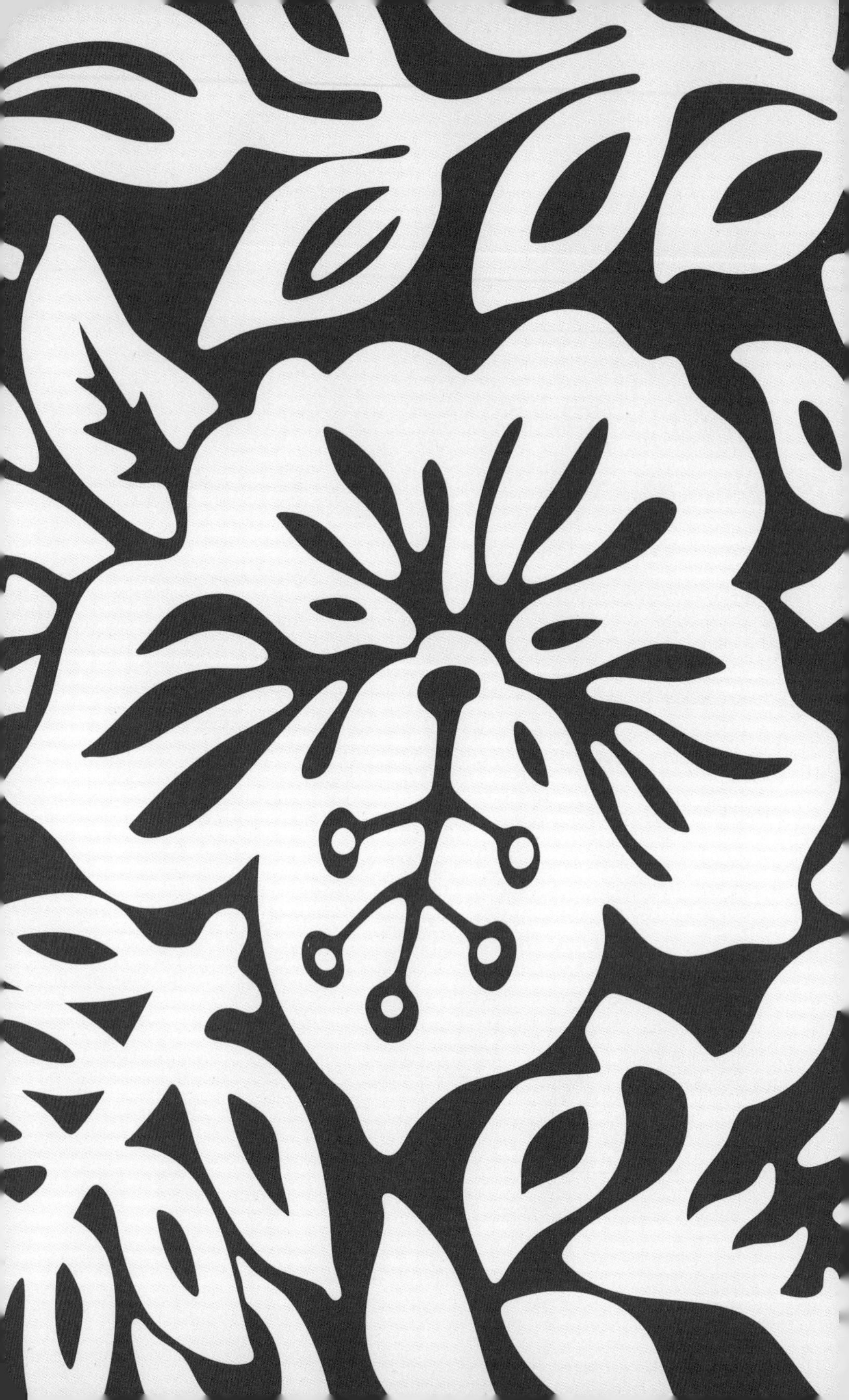

Month 5

Monthly check-in

Date: __________

Weeks of gestation: __________

Blood pressure: __________

Weight: __________

Fundal height: __________

Baby's heart rate: __________

What was the most exciting thing that happened this last month?

What was the funniest moment?

Cravings, body changes, and other monthly notes:

What questions do you have for your healthcare professional?

Week 17

Baby brain

You may have experienced instances of forgetfulness or the ability to think straight. Maybe you've left your car keys in the refrigerator or forgotten why you walked into a room. These instances can be both funny and sometimes frustrating. And many people blame them on pregnancy. There isn't enough information to support the existence of *baby brain* — a term used to describe the idea that pregnancy can affect memory and the ability to think. Some studies have shown that memory is impaired during pregnancy and shortly afterward, possibly due to hormonal changes, sleep deprivation or the stress of coping with a major life change. However, other research has shown that pregnancy has no negative cognitive impacts.

Have you noticed any changes in your ability to think or your memory? Have you blamed them on baby brain? How might the emotional and physical transitions of pregnancy be affecting you? What practical strategies can you use to reassure yourself or manage any changes to your memory?

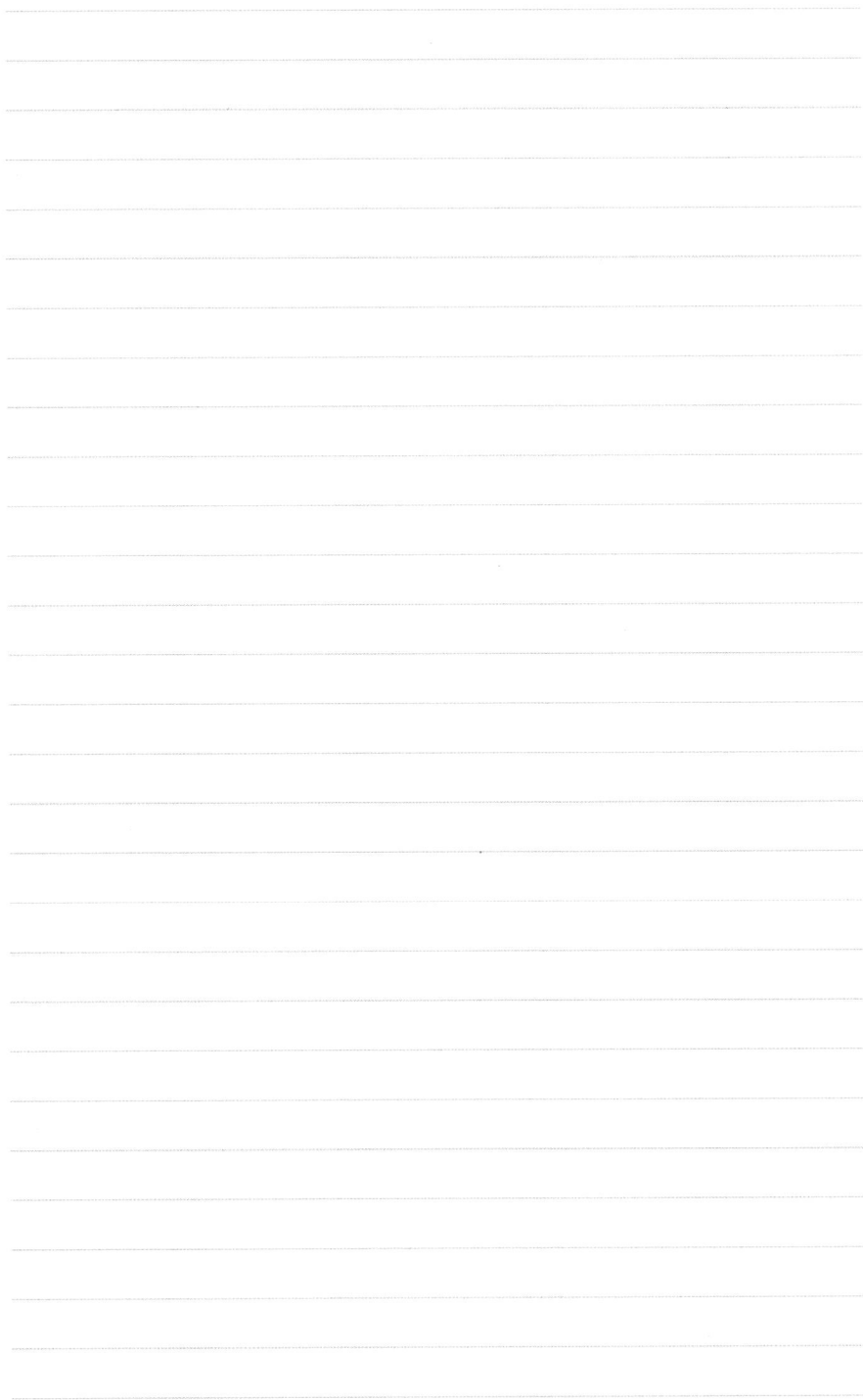

Week 18

Baby on the move!

The fifth month may bring an exciting milestone. Not only is your tummy continuing to grow in size, you may even start to feel your baby move. That's really your child in there!

Feeling your baby flip, kick or punch for the first time — usually around the 20th week of pregnancy — is a great source of wonder and reassurance for most people. In time, your partner will be able to feel baby's movements, too, by placing a hand on your abdomen. If you can't feel baby move yet, don't worry — those fluttering first movements will come soon. Depending on the position of your placenta, you may not feel kicks for a few more weeks.

Can you feel baby move yet? If not, come back to this when you do. What does it feel like? Does this bring relief, excitement or something else?

By this week, the bones in your baby's inner ear are developed enough to function, and nerve endings from the brain are hooked up to the ears. This means baby can now hear sounds.

As hearing continues to develop, baby will become familiar with the sounds and voices heard most over the next few months. What activities, such as talking to baby or playing them music, might you do to increase your bond?

Week 19

Your body changes: Reaching the midway point

You're halfway there! As you reach the midway point of pregnancy, your uterus will expand to your navel. Your pregnancy may now be quite obvious.

This month, you may notice that your breasts have become larger, with more visible veins. You may feel round ligament pain such as a sharp, jabbing pain in your lower abdomen or groin. Shortness of breath is also common.

What new body changes have arisen over the last month?
What strategies can you use to cope with problematic symptoms?
Do you have any concerns to bring up with your healthcare team?

Did you know?

Your baby can now swallow and may make conscious movements such as sucking a thumb or moving their head.

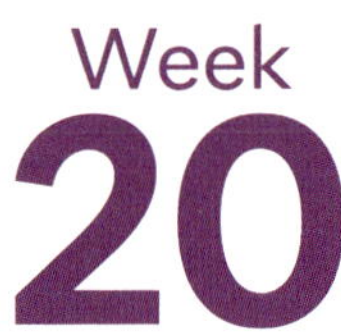

Week 20

Ultrasound and baby's sex

Most parents have an ultrasound around 18 to 20 weeks. This is an exciting benchmark for many parents, as the professional doing the scan may be able to tell your baby's sex, depending on baby's position. (If you want to keep that information a surprise, remember to give your care team a heads-up!) During the ultrasound, your baby's anatomy and heart rate and the amount of amniotic fluid will also be evaluated.

If you'd like, tape or glue a copy of your ultrasound picture below. (The pocket inside the back cover can hold additional photos.) Add any notes you may want on memorable observations that were made and on any measurements or stats taken during the ultrasound.

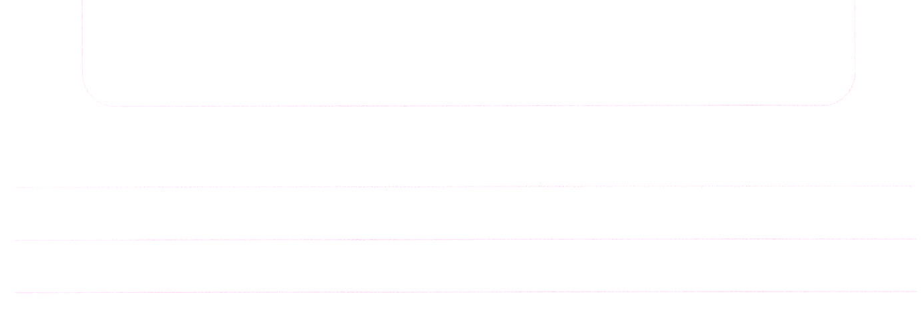

If you had an ultrasound this month, what was it like? What new information did you learn about your baby's health? How do you feel about this information?

Did you learn your baby's sex? If so, are you having a boy or a girl? If you hadn't already learned this news, how do you feel about it? Does knowing your baby's sex affect the way you're preparing for their arrival?

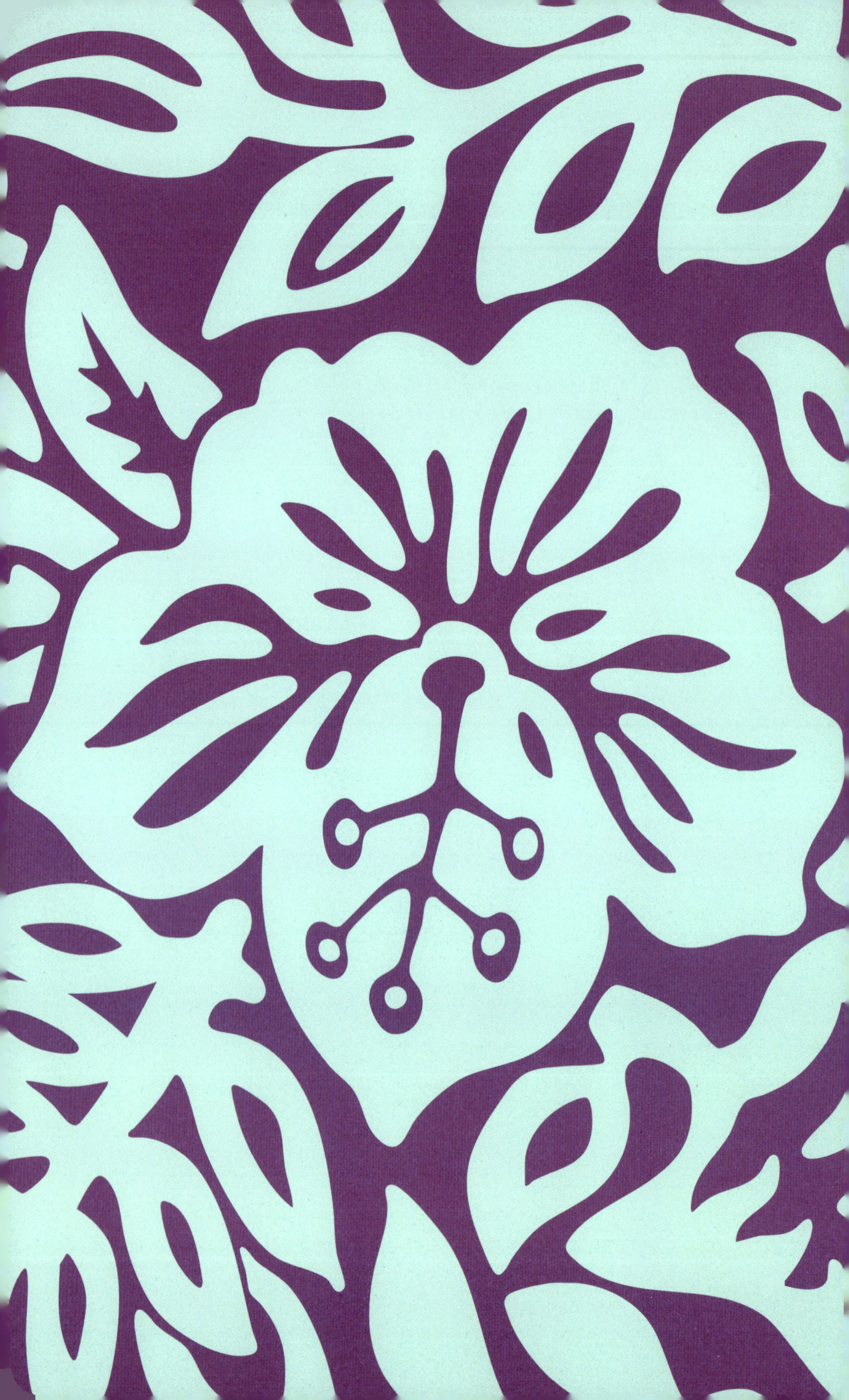

Month 6

Monthly check-in

Date:

Weeks of gestation:

Blood pressure:

Weight:

Fundal height:

Baby's heart rate:

What was the most exciting thing that happened this last month?

What was the funniest moment?

Cravings, body changes, and other monthly notes:

What questions do you have for your healthcare professional?

Week 21

Have no fear!

You and your partner may be worrying about the process of giving birth. Having some fear about the big day is understandable — but not to worry! There are many different ways you can work to relieve or confront your fears. Becoming knowledgeable through childbirth classes, practicing relaxation techniques and finding coping strategies can go a long way in keeping those fears in check. You can start by familiarizing yourself with the stages of labor (see page 130). You might also look into hiring a doula or other birth coach to help you through the process. Even something as simple as writing and sharing your fears with your partner and healthcare team can help you feel better.

What concerns or fears do you have about labor and delivery? What concerns or fears does your partner have? How do your fears compare? What does your healthcare team have to say about your concerns?

Did you know?

Your baby is developing their sense of taste and touch! They can now start to feel their face and touch other parts of their body.

Sharing intimacy with your partner

If you're like many people, you may be more interested in sex now than you were earlier in your pregnancy — and perhaps even more than you were before you became pregnant! Of course, this isn't universal, and it's possible you may not feel it at all.

How has your interest in sex changed over the course of your pregnancy? How has your partner's interest in sex been affected? Have these changes affected your relationship? What can you do to maintain your relationship if your levels of desire are mismatched?

Week

22

Good to know: What are hypertensive disorders?

Preeclampsia is a disorder specific to pregnancy and is marked by high blood pressure and protein in the urine after the 20th week of pregnancy. Preeclampsia affects 5% to 8% of all pregnancies and occurs most often during a person's first pregnancy. Preeclampsia should be treated as soon as possible as it can be dangerous for you and baby if left untreated.

People may have preeclampsia for several weeks before signs and symptoms develop. Headaches, vision problems and pain in the upper abdomen are other common symptoms of preeclampsia.

Have you been diagnosed with preeclampsia or has your care team had concerns about your blood pressure? If so, what instructions have you been given for managing the hypertension? How are you feeling about these changes?

If you don't have a diagnosis but are concerned you may have preeclampsia or hypertension, contact your healthcare team right away.

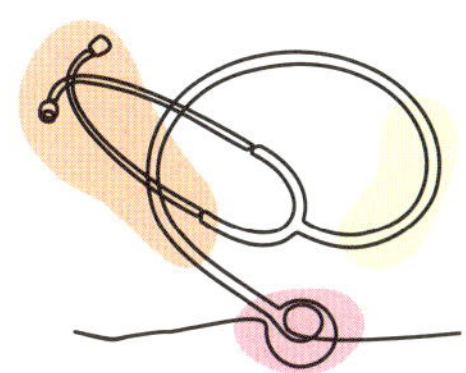

Thinking ahead: Finding healthcare for your baby

It's a good idea to decide who you want to provide healthcare to your baby before your child is born. This can be a family physician, pediatrician, nurse practitioner or physician assistant. Your baby will most likely have their first checkup within a week of being born. Having a healthcare professional picked out can make this process much easier. It also means you'll have someone you can call with any questions regarding newborn care. This can be very helpful and reassuring if you, like most first-time parents, have many questions.

What type of professional would you like your child to see? What qualifications and bedside manner would help you trust that person with your child's care? Do they need to have a certain level of accessibility or be in a certain insurance network? What other factors are important to you in making your decision? Could you ask your current healthcare team, family, friends, colleagues or neighbors for referrals or suggestions?

Did you know?

By the end of the month, your baby will start getting a sense of whether they are upside down or right side up inside your uterus. That's because your baby's inner ear, which controls balance in the body, will be developed.

Week 23

Your body changes: Feel those kicks!

Your baby's kicks may be much stronger than last month. They may even be strong enough for your partner and loved ones to feel.

As baby grows this month, you may experience hemorrhoids, hip pain, urine leaks, vulvar varicosities (varicose veins) and vaginal prolapse. Your breasts may even start making colostrum (see the Did you know? box on the next page).

What new body changes have arisen over the last month?
What strategies can you use to cope with problematic symptoms?
Do you have any concerns to bring up with your healthcare team?

Did you know?

You may start noticing droplets of watery or yellowish fluid appearing on your nipples, even this early. This early milk is called colostrum and is loaded with active, infection-fighting antibodies. If you choose to breastfeed, colostrum will be your baby's food for the first few days after birth.

Your body changes: Braxton Hicks contractions

Around this time, you may experience warm-up contractions called Braxton Hicks contractions. Try not to panic — these aren't actual contractions. They may feel like a painless squeezing sensation near the top of your uterus or in your lower abdomen and groin. Have you had any Braxton Hicks contractions? What did they feel like? How did you respond?

Contact your healthcare team if you're having contractions that concern you, especially if they become painful or if you have more than six in an hour.

Week 24

Childbirth classes

It's a good time to sign up for childbirth classes if this is your first pregnancy — or even if it's not but you want additional support in preparing for labor and delivery. Such classes are available at most hospitals and birthing centers, so ask about them at one of your prenatal visits. They may even have free resources you can take advantage of.

You and your partner will likely learn about signs of labor, pain relief options during labor, birthing positions and postnatal care. Some classes teach about caring for a newborn, including information on breastfeeding. You'll also learn about what will happen to your body during labor and birth, which can help you feel empowered rather than fearful about the process. (In fact, there are proven benefits to reducing fear of childbirth!) Some childbirth classes teach specific methods, such as Lamaze, Bradley and Mindfulness-Based Childbirth and Parenting (MBCP). There are also classes on specific topics, such as vaginal birth after C-section (VBAC). If this is not your first pregnancy, there may also be childbirth refresher courses available.

If you've signed up for a childbirth class, how did you choose it? If you haven't, what methods or topics interest you?

Choosing a childbirth class

Look for a class taught by a certified childbirth educator. This may be a nurse, midwife or other certified professional. The classes should be small, with no more than 8 to 10 couples, to facilitate discussion and allow for personalized instruction. The classes should also be comprehensive, addressing all aspects of labor and delivery, as well as newborn care. Be sure to ask about the cost as well. In addition, first-time parents may want to look for separate classes or clinics that offer more detailed information on topics that will be helpful after baby arrives. Check for classes near you on baby care basics, breastfeeding and car seat safety and installation.

Some common types of childbirth classes include:

- *Lamaze:* The goal of Lamaze is to increase confidence in your ability to give birth. Lamaze classes help you understand how to cope with pain in ways that both facilitate labor and promote comfort.
- *Bradley:* The Bradley Method emphasizes that birth is a natural process. You're taught to manage labor through deep breathing, a variety of relaxation techniques and the support of your partner or labor coach.
- *Mindfulness-Based Childbirth and Parenting (MBCP):* As the name implies, this newer method is driven by the concept of mindfulness — paying attention in the present moment without judgment.
- *Alternative approaches to childbirth:* These include hypnotherapy and water birth.

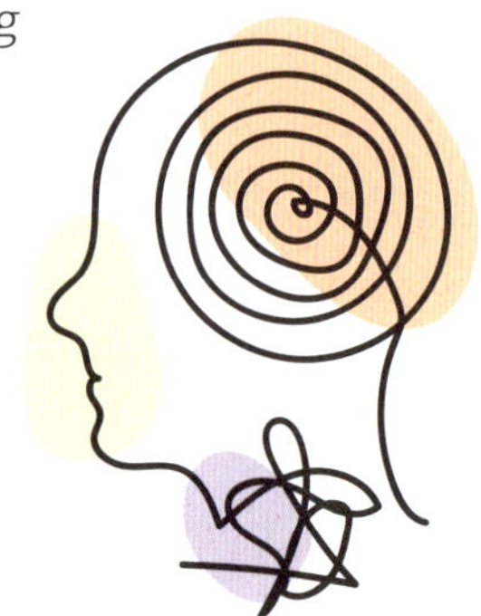

What are you hoping to get out of your childbirth classes?

Good to know: Learning about glucose testing and gestational diabetes

Usually sometime between weeks 24 through 28 of your pregnancy, you'll have a glucose test. This tests for gestational diabetes, a form of diabetes that can appear during pregnancy. If you have certain risk factors, your healthcare team may have you do the test earlier. Depending on the results, you may need to return for a second test.

It's important to know that while you can reduce certain risk factors, gestational diabetes can develop in anyone and in any pregnancy. So if you are diagnosed, know that it's not your fault. Hormones change how your body uses insulin during pregnancy. But in some people, the body can't make enough insulin to compensate and keep blood sugar levels in a normal range.

If you are diagnosed with gestational diabetes, you'll need to carefully control your blood glucose levels for the remainder of your pregnancy. This will include daily blood sugar monitoring. Most people with well-controlled gestational diabetes have healthy pregnancies and healthy babies. However, gestational diabetes that is not carefully managed can cause problems for both you and baby.

Have you done glucose testing yet? What was the experience like? If you had to return for a second test, how did it go? If you've been diagnosed with gestational diabetes, are you comfortable with the changes you need to make to your lifestyle? Do you have family, friends or other resources that you can reach out to for support?

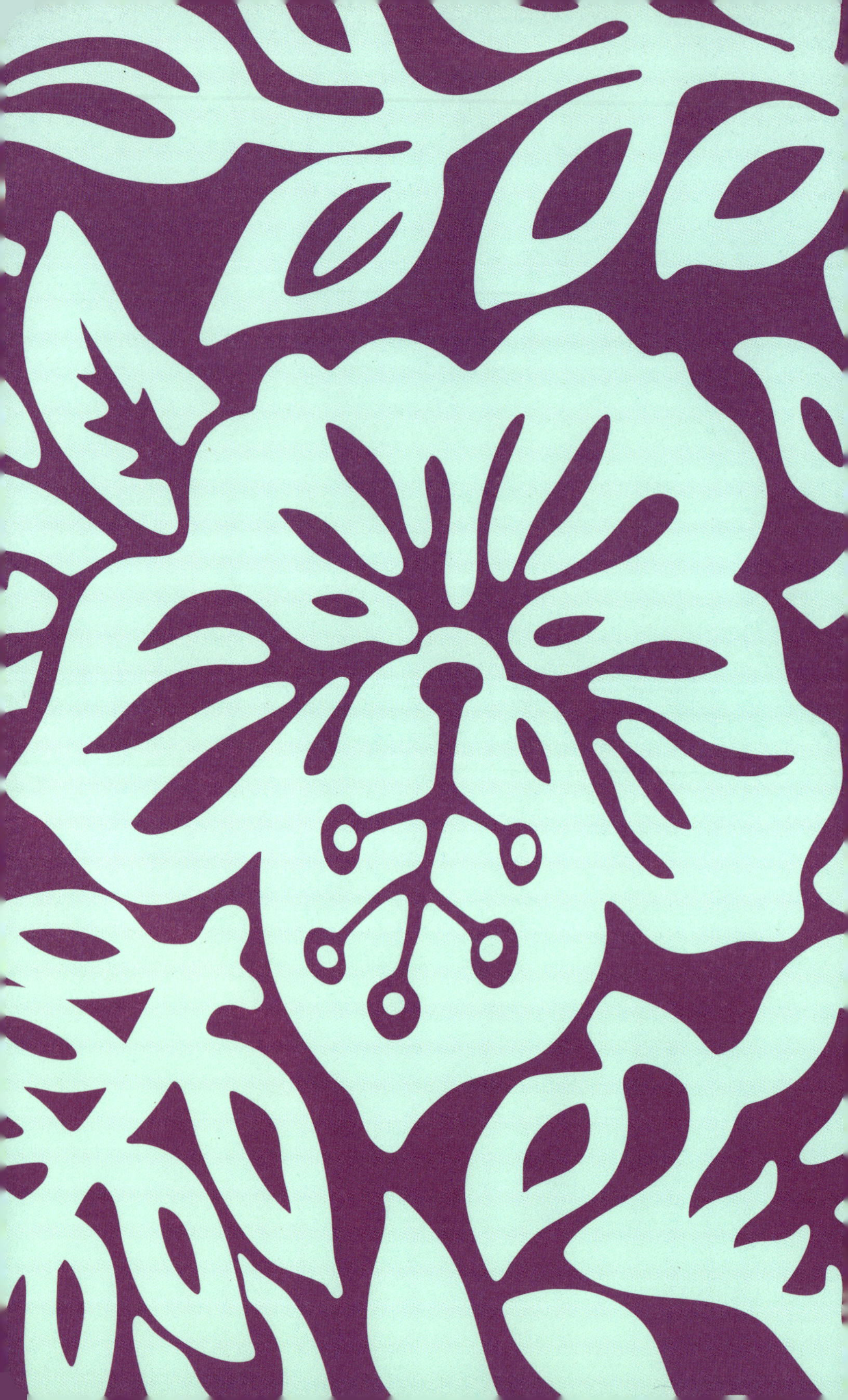

Month 7

Monthly check-in

Date:

Weeks of gestation:

Blood pressure:

Weight:

Fundal height:

Baby's heart rate:

What was the most exciting thing that happened this last month?

What was the funniest moment?

Cravings, body changes, and other monthly notes:

What questions do you have for your healthcare professional?

Week

25

Enjoy a little break

Slow down, sit back and relax. Try to enjoy this month of your pregnancy before the last preparations and discomforts of the final months begin. You might want to enjoy a low-key getaway or complete a small project at home — and make sure you're in photos from this time.

What would it look like for you to enjoy this month of your pregnancy? How can you revel in the emotions and sensations of being pregnant? What activities can you do to make the most of this time of the pregnancy?

Preparing your body for late pregnancy

Add these exercises to your routine. They can help strengthen and prepare the muscles that will receive the most stress in late pregnancy and delivery.

Kegel exercises: The muscles in your pelvic floor help support your uterus, bladder and bowel. Toning them by doing Kegel exercises will help ease your discomfort during the last months of your pregnancy.

How to do it. Identify your pelvic floor muscles — the muscles around your vagina and anus. When you finish urinating, stay sitting on the toilet. Imagine "closing" your vagina or that you are stopping gas from passing. You can also place a finger in your vagina and squeeze the vaginal muscles around it. When you contract your pelvic floor muscles in this way, you are doing a Kegel. To make sure you've found the right muscles, you can try to stop the flow of urine while you're going to the bathroom. Don't make this a habit, though. Doing Kegel exercises while urinating or when your bladder is full can be confusing to your body and lead to problems with emptying your bladder.

Perineal massage: Massaging the area between your vaginal opening and anus (perineum) in the last weeks before labor may help stretch these tissues in preparation for childbirth.

How to do it. Make sure your nails are trimmed. Wash your hands thoroughly with soap and hot water. Then put a mild lubricant on your thumbs and insert them inside your vagina. Press downward toward the rectum, stretching the tissues. Repeat daily for about 8 to 10 minutes. Your partner can help with this process, if you wish. You may experience a little burning or other discomfort as you massage your perineum. This is normal. However, stop if you begin to feel sharp pain.

Week 26

Your baby's growth: Second trimester

This month, your little boy or girl will do most of their growing before they enter the world. They will add more body fat, which will make their skin look more smooth and less wrinkled. The skin will also begin to take on a little more color. Your baby's eyebrows and eyelashes are now well formed, and more hair has grown on their head. Your baby's footprints and fingerprints are now formed. And all the components that make up the eyes have developed, though your baby probably won't open their eyes for about two more weeks. By 26 weeks, your baby weighs between 1 ½ and 2 pounds.

Is baby's development in line with what you expected by this time? Does learning about baby's growth make you relate differently to your baby or your body?

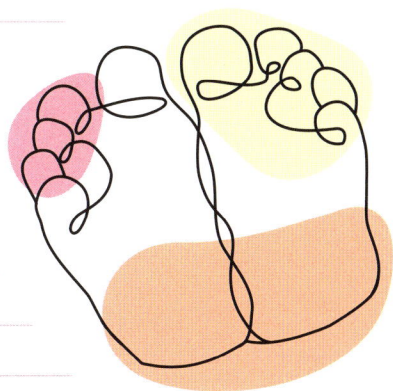

Week 27

Breastfeeding, formula-feeding or both?

The decision to use breast milk or formula — or a combination of both — is a personal one. Some people know right from the start what they'll do, while others struggle with the decision. If you haven't come to a decision already, it's probably time to think about how you plan to feed your baby. Breast milk and formula can both give your baby the nutrients needed to grow and be perfectly healthy, and allow for precious bonding time together.

The benefits of breastfeeding — whether by directly breastfeeding, pumping or both — are well established. In fact, breastfeeding has numerous benefits for both you and baby. The American Academy of Pediatrics recommends that infants be fed breast milk exclusively for the first six months. However, a wide range of factors may lead you to consider formula-feeding. For people deciding between methods of feeding, the best thing to do is learn about all of them and then take comfort in knowing that you made an informed decision.

Have you decided what method or combination of methods you want to use? If so, how did you come to your decision? What hopes do you have for feeding your baby? What concerns do you have? If you haven't decided yet, what factors are you considering? Where can you learn more about the different methods? Who can help you make your decision?

Can't decide? Try this!

Try talking with your healthcare team, family and friends. They may offer recommendations or advice to help you decide. Some respected websites, such as HealthyChildren.org and La Leche League, also offer resources and support. If you're still undecided about what to do, here's a suggestion: Give breastfeeding a try. Make it part of your birth plan so that you'll receive breastfeeding support after you deliver. Consider asking your healthcare team for a lactation consultant referral. This specialist may provide additional support if you need it after returning home.

Week 28

Protecting your personal space

When you're visibly pregnant, everyone from relatives to complete strangers may believe it's OK to comment on your body or even touch your belly. Additionally, people may tell you about difficult pregnancy, childbirth and postpartum experiences they or a friend of theirs had. This often comes from an intent to connect with you.

Still, pregnant or not, you get to determine who's allowed to touch your body. For example, you can say "please stop," or "I prefer that people not touch my belly." In the moment, stepping back and covering your own belly with your hands can also help send that message. You might also consider verbal and nonverbal cues you might use to set boundaries about the information and types of comments you engage with.

How have your boundaries been respected or disregarded during your pregnancy? How would you prefer to respond if someone attempts to cross a boundary or talk about something you don't feel comfortable with?

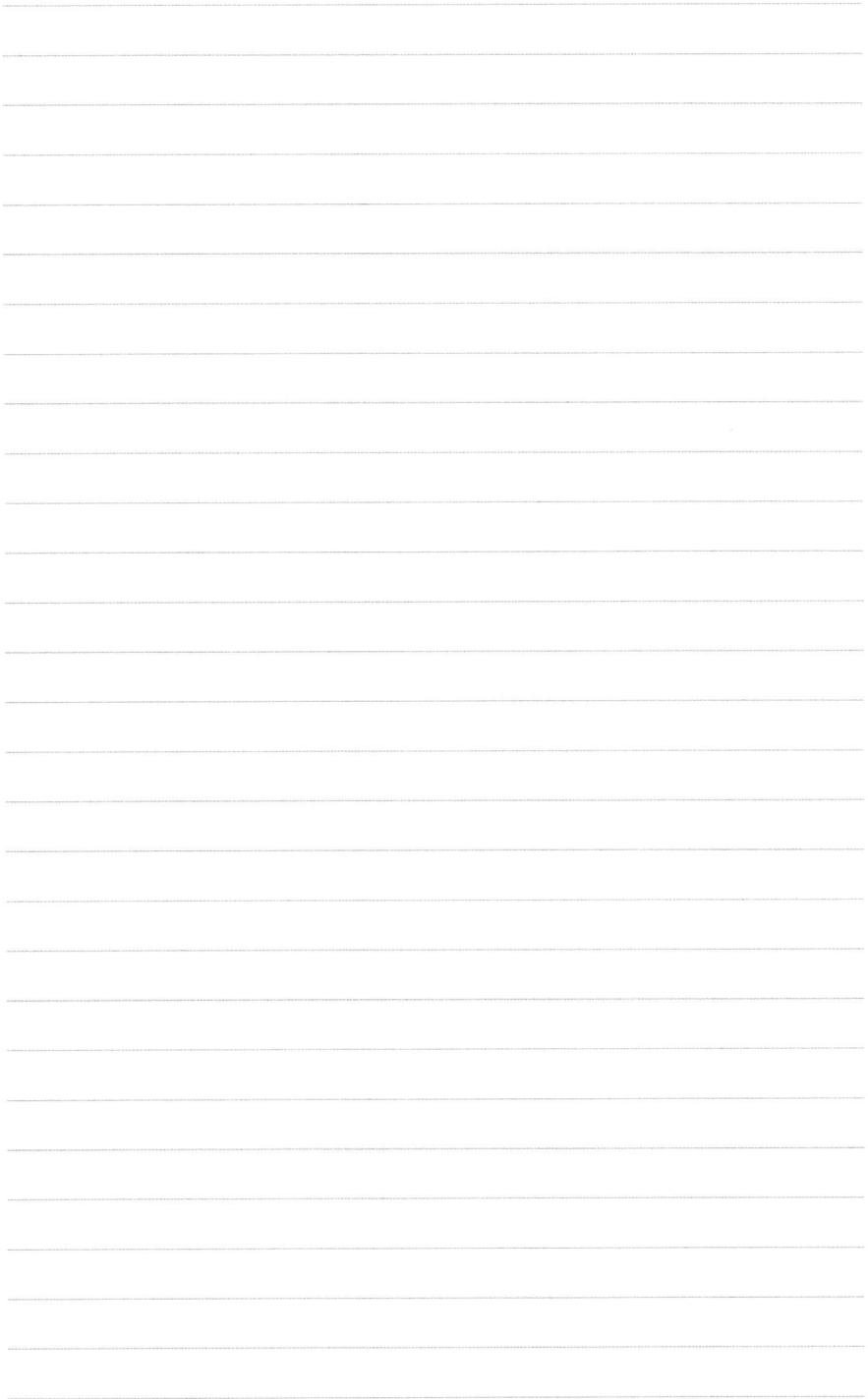

Your body changes: Bigger belly, bigger baby

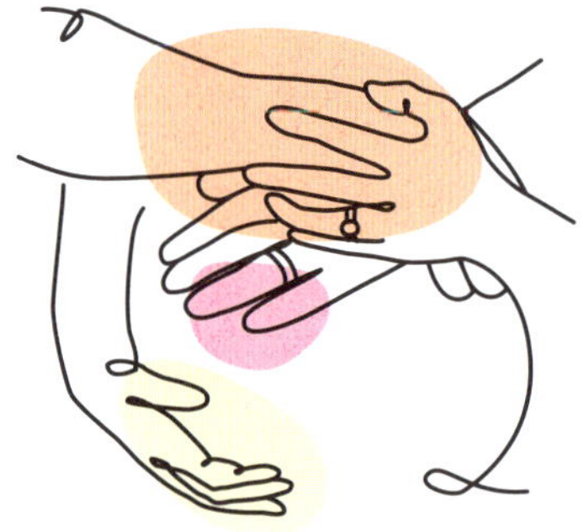

As you watch your belly get bigger, you may wonder if there's any room left for your baby to grow more. (Spoiler: There is!) As your uterus expands further upward, your baby will become increasingly active.

New body changes this month may include bumps around your areolas, pelvic pain and spider veins. You may also feel heart palpitations. This sensation usually doesn't signify anything serious. But if you experience this feeling, tell your healthcare team, especially if you also have chest pain or shortness of breath.

What new body changes have you noticed over the last month? What strategies can you use to cope with problematic symptoms? Do you have any concerns to bring up with your healthcare team?

Did you know?

For many babies, their most active time is between 27 and 32 weeks. They are now big enough to pack a punch, and they still have room to do so.

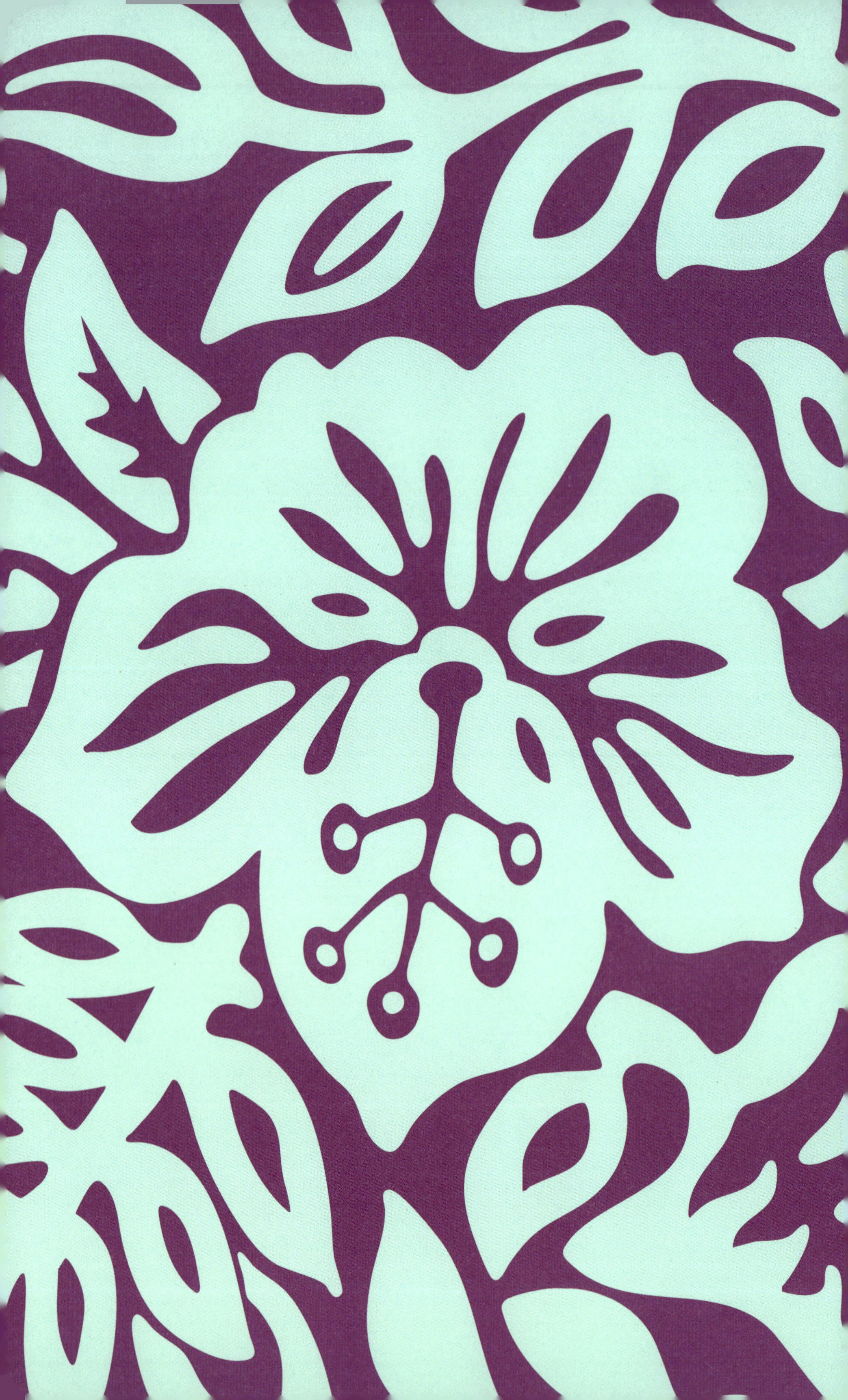

Month 8

Monthly check-in

Date:

Weeks of gestation:

Blood pressure:

Weight:

Fundal height:

Baby's heart rate:

What was the most exciting thing that happened this last month?

What was the funniest moment?

Cravings, body changes, and other monthly notes:

What questions do you have for your healthcare professional?

Week 29

Managing anxiety

In just a few months, you'll be responsible for a new human being. It might be scary to think about, but you can do this!

To help keep anxiety at bay, review some of the decisions that need to be made before your baby is born. Is your baby going to see a pediatrician or a family doctor? Are you going to feed your baby with breast milk or formula? If your baby is a boy, are you going to have his penis circumcised? What other decisions have you made? Taking stock of where you stand on these issues will help you feel more in control of the situation.

If you feel like anxiety is interfering with your daily life, talk to your care team. Help is available, and caring for your mental health is important as you approach this transition.

Have you experienced more anxiety recently? How has anxiety affected your daily life and your sleep? What relaxation exercises can you do to reduce your anxiety? (See week 37 for more information on relaxation and calming techniques.)

Did you know?

From now until delivery, your baby will gain about half a pound a week!

Third trimester to-do list:

Things to consider as you enter your third trimester. Continue reading to learn more about some of these tasks. You can also fill in the blank spaces with any additional items you want to consider.

- ☐ Schedule follow-up prenatal appointments
- ☐ Start buying baby gear
- ☐ Create a birth plan
- ☐ Prepare for labor and childbirth
- ☐ Pack your hospital bag
- ☐ Do your group B strep test
- ☐ Get vaccinated per your healthcare team's recommendations (RSV, Tdap)

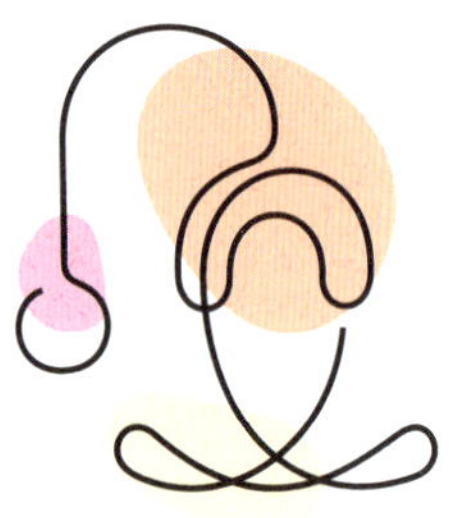

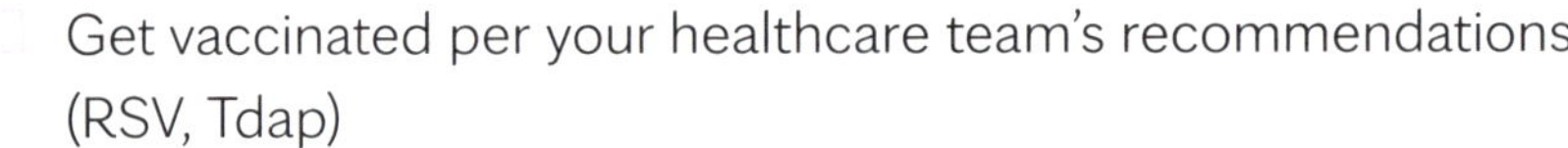

Week 30

Baby gear essentials

As you approach your baby's due date, it's time to go gear shopping. You'll want to give extra consideration to a car seat, crib, carrier and stroller. For these items especially, safety is key. Research safety information and product details before making your purchase. Make sure you're purchasing baby gear that will fit your needs and that's designed to keep your baby as safe as possible. For more information on making safe baby gear purchases, see ***Mayo Clinic Guide to a Healthy Pregnancy.***

What baby gear have you purchased, registered for or received already? How did you decide on what to buy for bigger purchases? What safety information do you still need to review? What makes you excited about these purchases? What worries and concerns do you have about them?

Baby gear checklist

Deciding what kind of gear to get can be challenging — but also a lot of fun! Consider your practical needs and, as your budget allows, the styles or features that you'd like. Here is a basic checklist with items to consider getting for you and your baby:

Bathtime

- [ ] baby bathtub
- [ ] baby-safe shampoo or bodywash
- [ ] towels
- [ ] washcloths
- [ ] ______
- [ ] ______
- [ ] ______
- [ ] ______
- [ ] ______
- [ ] ______
- [ ] ______
- [ ] ______
- [ ] ______
- [ ] ______
- [ ] ______
- [ ] ______

Diapering

- [ ] diapers
- [ ] wipes
- [ ] diaper pail
- [ ] diaper rash cream
- [ ] ______
- [ ] ______
- [ ] ______
- [ ] ______
- [ ] ______
- [ ] ______
- [ ] ______
- [ ] ______
- [ ] ______
- [ ] ______
- [ ] ______
- [ ] ______
- [ ] ______

Clothes

- [ ] swaddle blankets and sleep sacks
- [ ] onesies and bodysuits
- [ ] socks and booties
- [ ] footed pajamas
- [ ] pants and shorts
- [ ] hats
- [ ] long-sleeved and short-sleeved shirts
- [ ] sweaters and jackets
- [ ] snowsuit and fleece bunting (if needed)
- [ ] ______
- [ ] ______
- [ ] ______
- [ ] ______
- [ ] ______
- [ ] ______
- [ ] ______
- [ ] ______
- [ ] ______
- [ ] ______

Feeding

- [ ] bottles
- [ ] bottle and nipple brush
- [ ] breast pads and nipple cream
- [ ] breast pump and extra parts
- [ ] milk storage containers or freezer bags
- [ ] nursing pillow
- [ ] burp cloths
- [ ] formula
- [ ] bibs
- [ ] high chair
- [ ] kid-friendly plates, bowls, sippy cups, feeding spoons
- [ ] ______
- [ ] ______
- [ ] ______
- [ ] ______
- [ ] ______
- [ ] ______
- [ ] ______

Health and Safety

- [ ] baby first aid kit
- [ ] bulb syringe or nasal aspirator
- [ ] nail clippers and file
- [ ] thermometer
- [ ] outlet covers
- [ ] baby gates
- [ ]
- [ ]
- [ ]
- [ ]
- [ ]
- [ ]
- [ ]
- [ ]
- [ ]
- [ ]
- [ ]
- [ ]
- [ ]
- [ ]

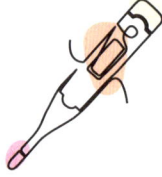

Travel

- [ ] car seat with base
- [ ] diaper bag
- [ ] stroller
- [ ] baby sun hats
- [ ] baby-safe sunscreen (not recommended for use until six months)
- [ ] cooler bag for bottles or food
- [ ]
- [ ]
- [ ]
- [ ]
- [ ]
- [ ]
- [ ]
- [ ]
- [ ]
- [ ]
- [ ]
- [ ]
- [ ]

Nursery

- [ ] crib
- [ ] crib mattress
- [ ] crib sheets
- [ ] waterproof mattress protectors

Other

Week 31

Your body changes: Continuing to grow

This month, your uterus will continue to expand toward the bottom of your rib cage, creating a new set of physical changes and symptoms. New body changes may include carpal tunnel syndrome, itchy or dry skin, low back and pubic symphysis pain, puffiness and swelling, sciatica and stretch marks. You might also find that you get tired more easily. On the other hand, you may also notice that your hair is fuller and healthier looking. This may last for a few weeks or months postpartum.

What new body changes have arisen over the last month? What strategies can you use to cope with problematic symptoms? Do you have any concerns to bring up with your healthcare team?

Did you know?

Normally, hair on your scalp grows about a half inch each month for 2 to 7 years. It then goes into a resting phase, stops growing and eventually falls out. During pregnancy, thanks to hormonal changes, your hair tends to remain in the growing phase.

Week

32

Good to know: Thinking about perinatal depression and anxiety

As your due date approaches, it's a good time to pause again and assess your mental health. Depression and anxiety can be problems during pregnancy as well as postpartum. Stress, body changes, pregnancy complications and not having enough support may all contribute to developing a mood disorder. Consider the symptoms of depression and anxiety on the next page. Do you have any of these symptoms? When did they start? Have you brought them up with your healthcare team?

Symptoms of perinatal anxiety and depression can include: Sleep disturbances, impaired thinking or concentration, significant and unexplained weight gain or loss, agitation or slowed body movements, fatigue, low self-esteem, loss of interest in sex, thoughts of death, persistent worrying and a sense of impending danger.

If you've been diagnosed with perinatal depression or anxiety, what treatment have you received? How is it working? Talk to your healthcare team about any changes you think you may need to make.

Continue to discuss any symptoms with your healthcare team whether or not you have a diagnosis of depression and anxiety. Remember that treatment, including counseling and certain medications, is considered safe during pregnancy and breastfeeding.

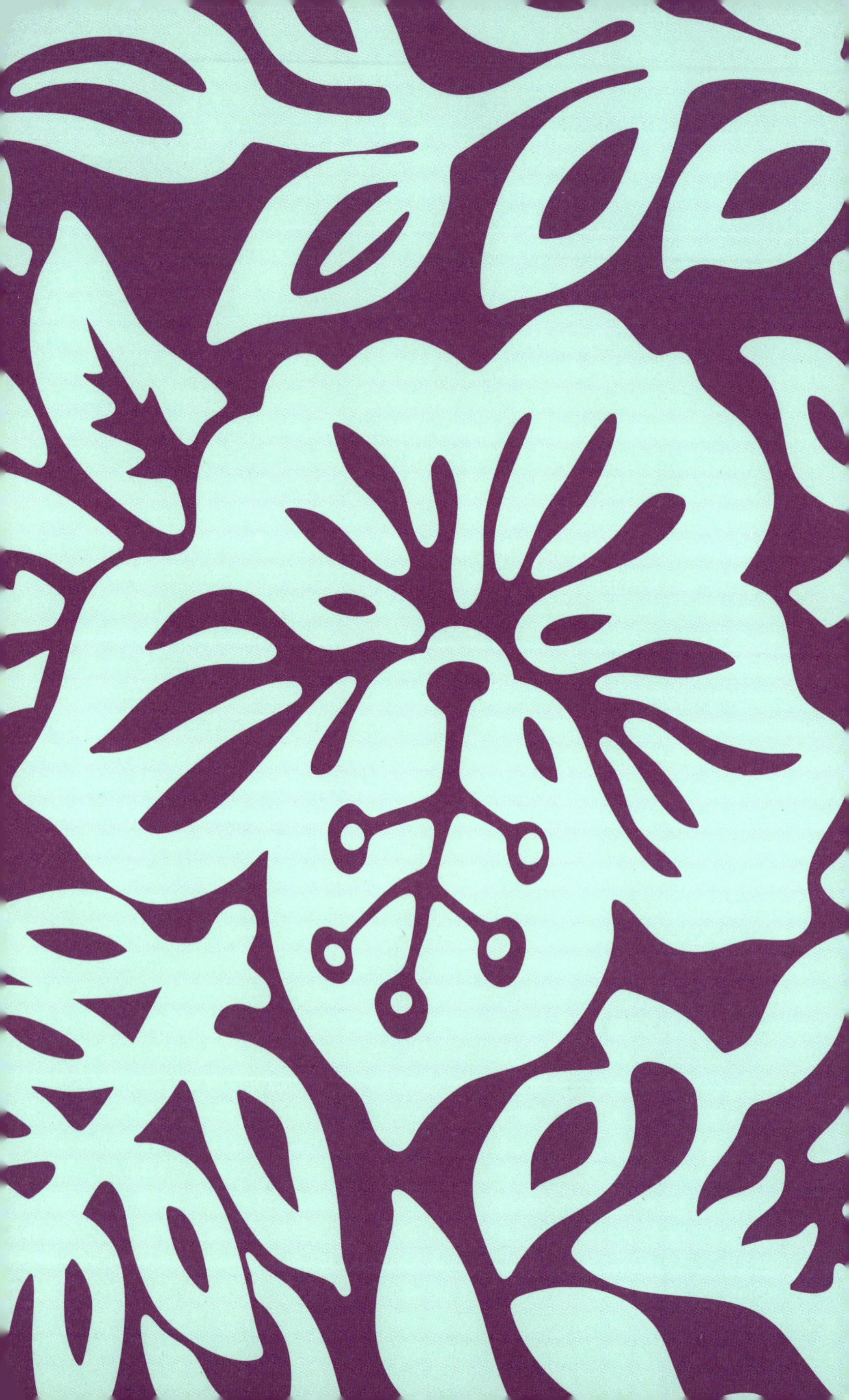

Month 9

Monthly check-in

Date:

Weeks of gestation:

Blood pressure:

Weight:

Fundal height:

Baby's heart rate:

What was the most exciting thing that happened this last month?

What was the funniest moment?

Cravings, body changes, and other monthly notes:

What questions do you have for your healthcare professional?

Week 33

Preparing yourself for labor

You're probably thinking a lot this month about when labor will start and how your childbirth experience will go. It's very common to feel anxious about labor and childbirth, especially if this is your first pregnancy.

To help you prepare and stay calm, be sure both you and your labor partner are educated through childbirth classes and books or other media from reliable sources. Review the overall process of labor that's outlined on page 130. In addition, try talking with people who have had positive birth experiences, familiarizing yourself with the various pain relief options available to you during labor, and telling yourself you'll do the best you can. If possible, talk to multiple people about what worked for them so you'll have a variety of tips to draw from. Hiring a doula or inquiring about doula services through your hospital and insurance may also help you feel ready for the big day.

Do you have different or new fears and anxieties about labor and childbirth? What questions do you still have about the process and the pain relief options available to you? Discuss those with your healthcare team at your next appointment. Who do you know that has had a positive childbirth experience? What tips have you learned after talking with others?

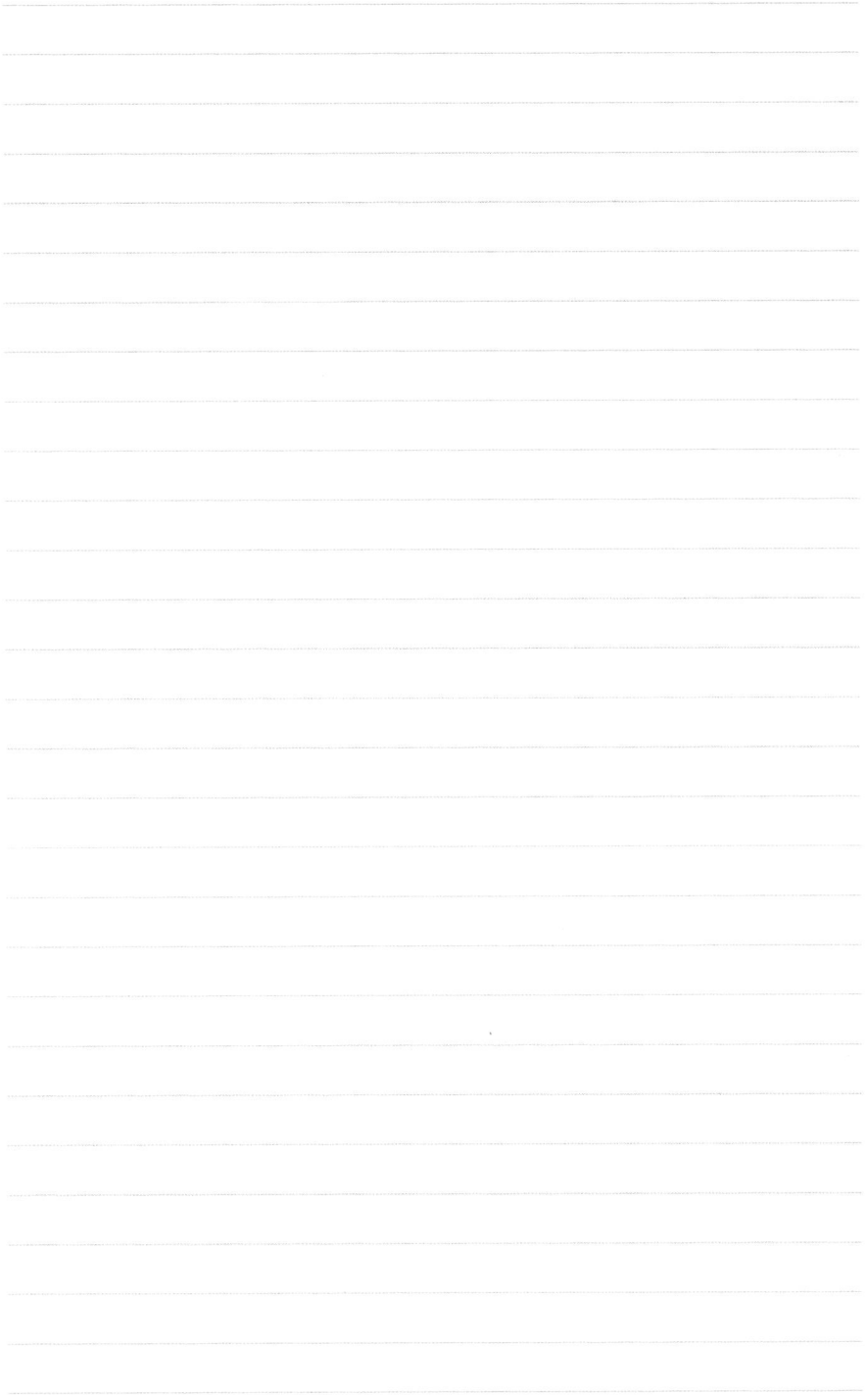

Week 34

Baby's position

During your visits this month, your healthcare professional will check baby's position. The position baby is in by the 33rd week of your pregnancy will likely be the position they will be in for delivery. If your baby is positioned headfirst, you're good to go. When the baby is positioned rump-first or feetfirst, they are in what's called a breech position, and your health professional may suggest a procedure to turn your baby.

What position was your baby in at your last prenatal visit? Were any procedures recommended to shift your baby's position? Can you tell what position your baby is in by how baby kicks or pokes? Can your partner see or feel these movements?

Did you know?

As baby grows bigger, you might be able to notice the shape of their elbow or heel against your abdomen.

Pain in the back

Backaches and back pain are common during pregnancy for several reasons. During pregnancy, the joints and ligaments in your pelvic region begin to soften and loosen in preparation for the baby to pass through your pelvis. As your uterus grows, your abdominal organs shift and your body weight is redistributed, changing your center of gravity. In response, you begin to adjust your posture and the ways you move. These compensations often lead to backaches and back pain.

Pain, tingling or numbness running down your buttock, back or thigh is called sciatica because it follows the course of the sciatic nerve, a major nerve that runs from your lower back down the back of your legs to your feet. Sciatica is caused by pressure on the sciatic nerve from your growing uterus or baby or by relaxed pelvic joints. Lifting, bending and even walking may aggravate sciatica.

Prevention and self-care: To prevent pain, practice good posture, tucking your pelvis under you when standing and pulling your shoulders back and down. Lift objects by squatting and lifting with your legs rather than bending over and lifting with your back. Avoid lifting heavy objects and avoid any sudden movements. Changing your position throughout the day, such as getting up and moving around every hour or so and not standing for a long time can prevent and relieve pain. Warm baths, a heating pad and switching the side of your body that you sleep on may help with back and leg pain. You can also try sleeping on your side with one or both knees bent and a pillow between your knees. Physical therapy or chiropractic care may also help relieve pain in the back and legs. Talk to your healthcare team if the pain becomes severe or if you're experiencing sciatic pain.

Your body changes: Fatigue and baby dropping (or not)

This month, your symptoms may vary depending on whether or not your baby has settled lower in your pelvis, or "dropped." Though this will bring more symptoms, you may find relief in the fact that your baby is getting ready to make their grand entrance!

This month, you might begin to notice new body changes such as increased vaginal discharge, loose-feeling limbs and sharp pain in the vagina. If your baby has dropped, you may also have improved heartburn and constipation, an easier time breathing and less sciatic pain.

What new body changes have arisen over the last month? Do you think your baby has dropped? How can you tell? Do you have any concerns to bring up with your healthcare team?

Week

35

Packing your hospital bag

Because your due date isn't a given, it's a good idea to have your bag packed and ready for the hospital or birth center ahead of time. If you don't want to put everything into your bag yet, make a list so that you can gather items easily when you prepare to leave. Your partner will also want to be prepared to stay with you, with their own clothes, snacks and toiletries set aside. In addition, have a car seat installed for baby's ride home.

What items do you still need to gather or prepare for your hospital bag? Is the car seat installed? Are you feeling prepared for baby's arrival?

Hospital bag checklist

Here are some items you may want to have on hand for the birth and the first days after:

- ☐ Copy of your birth preferences
- ☐ Nursing bra or, if you plan to bottle-feed, a supportive bra
- ☐ Phone with a camera, camera or video camera and charger
- ☐ Robe
- ☐ Comfortable clothes to wear at the hospital and loose clothing for going home — probably a mid-pregnancy outfit
- ☐ Pajamas or a nightgown that opens in the front to allow for easy breastfeeding
- ☐ Several pairs of underwear large enough to fit over maternity pads
- ☐ Socks or slippers — labor rooms are often kept cool
- ☐ Favorite snacks and drinks for your stay after baby arrives
- ☐ Glasses — you may have to remove your contact lenses
- ☐ Lip balm for dry lips
- ☐ Moisturizer, toothbrush and toothpaste, other toiletries and any cosmetics or self-care products you'll want
- ☐ Baby blanket
- ☐ Baby clothes, including a hat, and a seasonally appropriate going-home outfit
- ☐ ____________________
- ☐ ____________________
- ☐ ____________________

Week

36

Good to know: Group B strep test

At this point in your pregnancy, your healthcare team may screen you for group B streptococcus (GBS), if they haven't already done so. People who harbor GBS may pass the bacterium to their babies during labor and delivery. Newborns have a higher risk of complications from GBS because they don't yet have proper immunity. If GBS is found, your care team will likely give you antibiotics once you go into labor. This reduces the risk that your baby will acquire the bacterium.

Have you had a GBS test? If the test was positive, do you have any worries or concerns? Who can you discuss these worries with?

Your birth plan

If you haven't already started, now's the time to think about your options and preferences regarding labor, delivery and postpartum care. No one can predict how birth will go, and things may change. But creating a birth plan encourages you to consider all the decisions that may be involved, and it also allows you to talk about your preferences with your healthcare team. Take some time to reflect here on what you've done so far and how you feel. Then on the following pages, you can start getting into the details of your plan.

Have you started a birth plan yet? What decisions do you still need to make? Who can help you with your birth plan? How do you feel about your birth plan so far?

Your birth plan: Pain management

To help labor and delivery go as smoothly as possible, it's best to know what may help you handle the pain when it arrives. There are various options for controlling labor-related pain, including breathing and relaxation techniques, pain-relieving medications and a combination of options. Familiarize yourself with all of your options. While it's smart to have a plan, try to keep an open mind. It's impossible to know exactly what you'll need and what will work best as your labor progresses.

What pain-relief method or methods would you like to use? How can you best prepare to use that approach? If you aren't sure what method you'd prefer, who can you talk to for recommendations? How do you feel about the options available and your choice?

Your birth plan: Cesarean section

Cesarean delivery — commonly known as a C-section — is a surgical procedure used to deliver your baby through an incision in your abdomen, rather than vaginally. Some C-sections are planned. If you have serious health issues, are having multiple babies or have had a previous C-section, you may be having a planned C-section.

However, in many cases, the need for a cesarean birth doesn't become obvious until labor has already started. This could be because your labor isn't progressing normally, you have a placenta problem or there is an umbilical cord problem. You may also need a C-section if your baby has an abnormal heart rate pattern, is in a difficult or unideal position, is very large or has a health problem.

Talk to your healthcare team to find out what the protocol is for when a C-section is recommended and share any concerns you may have. Knowing what to expect can help you prepare if a C-section is necessary. You can learn more about C-sections and recovery on the Mayo Clinic website and in ***Mayo Clinic Guide to a Healthy Pregnancy.***

Are you planning a C-section? If not, what modifications do you need to make to your birth plan in case a C-section is needed? Have you talked with your healthcare team about when or why a C-section may be recommended? Do you feel your concerns are heard so that you can share in decision-making and trust their recommendation for you and baby when the time comes?

Your birth plan: Checklist

As you work on your birth plan, there are many things to consider. Your healthcare team or hospital may ask you to fill out a form stating your preferences. Or you may create a birth plan of your own or as part of your childbirth classes. If you don't have a birth plan, you can fill in the list on the following pages to get started.

In addition, you may inform your healthcare team about your preferences for procedures, such as avoiding episiotomy, which is an incision to widen the vaginal opening, or C-section birth. But ultimately, the clinical situation typically dictates what procedures are needed to keep you and baby safe. Your care team will ask for your consent before going forward with any procedure.

Use your birth plan to think about your preferences for various questions that may come up during labor and childbirth. What are your preferences? Why do you feel that way? What obstacles may come up preventing you from following those preferences? What can you do if those obstacles arise?

Your birth plan: Birth preferences

- ☐ Concerns you may have regarding giving birth:

- ☐ Things you look forward to during birth:

- ☐ Your support person during labor and delivery, and anyone else you'd like present for the birth:

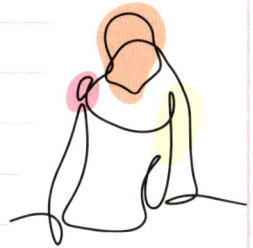

- ☐ Natural pain relief preferences:

- ☐ Pain medication preferences:

- [ ] Goals in terms of medication use:

- [ ] Hydration preferences:

- [ ] Positions for pushing and delivery:

- [ ] Preferences regarding the delivery, such as using a mirror:

- [ ] Preferences for photos or video:

- [ ] Preferences for what happens with your baby right after birth:

- [ ] Circumcision preference, if you have a boy:

- [ ] How you plan to feed your baby:

- [ ] Preferences regarding being present at the baby's first bath and exams:

- [ ] Parent and baby follow-up care:

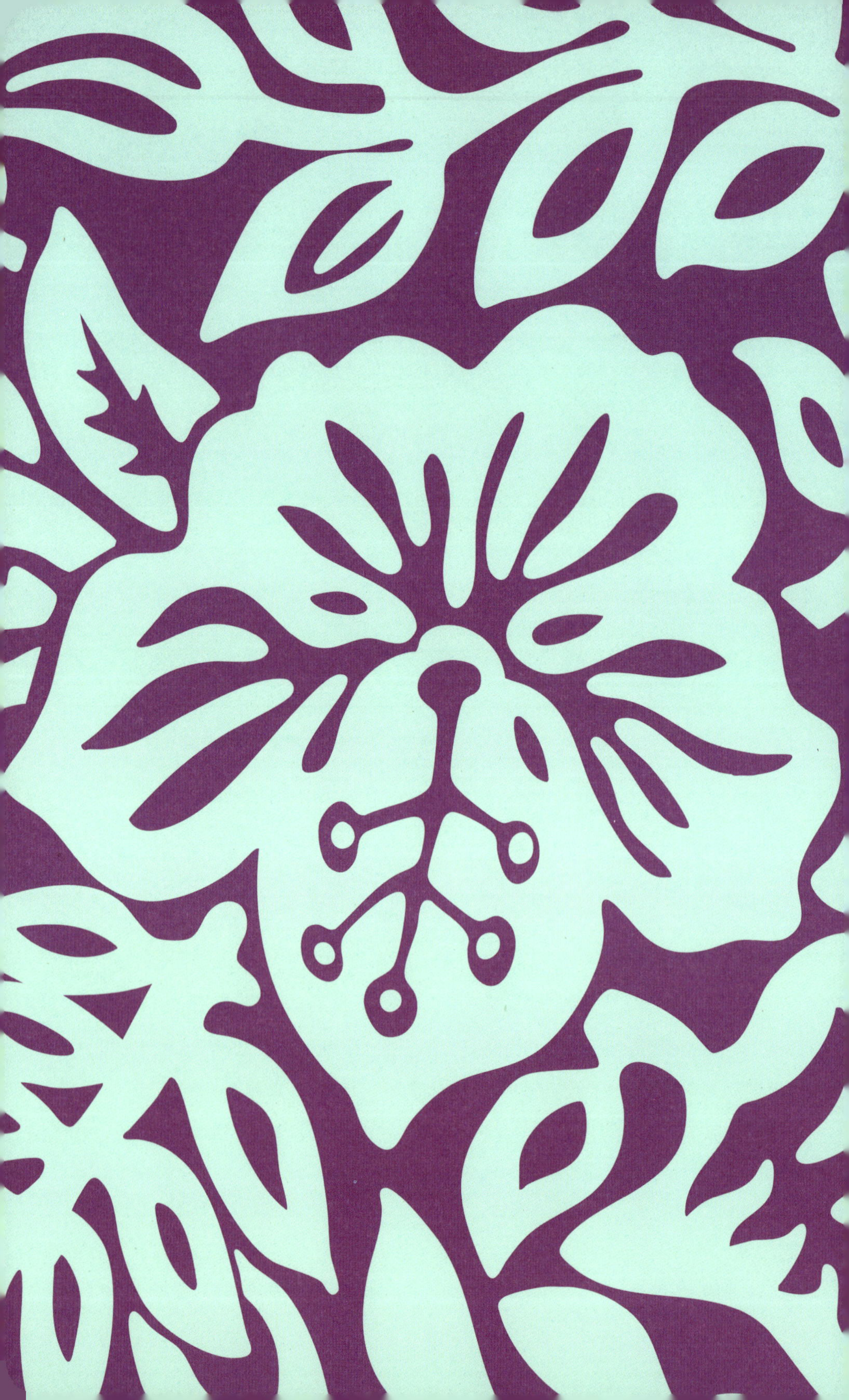

Month 10

Monthly check-in

Date: ______

Weeks of gestation: ______

Blood pressure: ______

Weight: ______

Fundal height: ______

Baby's heart rate: ______

What was the most exciting thing that happened this last month?

What was the funniest moment?

Cravings, body changes, and other monthly notes:

What questions do you have for your healthcare professional?

Week
37

Relaxation and calming techniques

Need a reason to take time out to relax? Practice makes perfect. If you're frightened and anxious during labor, you'll likely have a more difficult labor. Stress sets in motion a whole range of reactions in your body that can ultimately interfere with labor. Childbirth educators call it the fear-tension-pain cycle. To keep yourself from becoming too stressed, practice different ways of helping your body relax. These include progressive muscle relaxation, touch relaxation, massage, guided imagery, meditation and breathing techniques.

Try out different relaxation techniques. Which techniques do you like? Which seem the most effective? Can you envision using any of these techniques during labor? What would that look like? Who can help you to practice these techniques now and when you're in labor?

What are different relaxation techniques?

Progressive muscle relaxation: With this technique, you relax groups of muscles in a series when you feel yourself becoming tense. Beginning with your head or feet, relax one muscle group at a time, moving toward the other end of your body.

Touch relaxation: This is similar to progressive relaxation, but your cue for releasing each muscle group is when your labor coach presses on that area.

Massage: During labor, various massage techniques may help you relax.

Guided imagery: Sometimes called visualization, this involves imagining yourself in a comfortable and peaceful place, creating a feeling of relaxation and well-being.

Meditation: Focusing on a calming object, image or word can help you relax during labor and reduce the pain you experience.

Breathing techniques: Practiced, paced breathing activates your nervous system. This helps you relax and feel calm and can help reduce nausea and dizziness.

Week 38

Keeping busy

You're getting so close to the finish line! By this point, you may be having trouble sleeping. Time may seem to be standing still. Hang in there! To manage the anticipation and discomfort, try to stay busy. Keeping your mind active will help the days move more quickly until you're finally in labor.

What essentials can you check off your to-do list in preparation for your baby's arrival? What work do you need to complete before going on leave? Who do you want to spend time with? What are some hobbies or activities you can do to relax and get your mind off things?

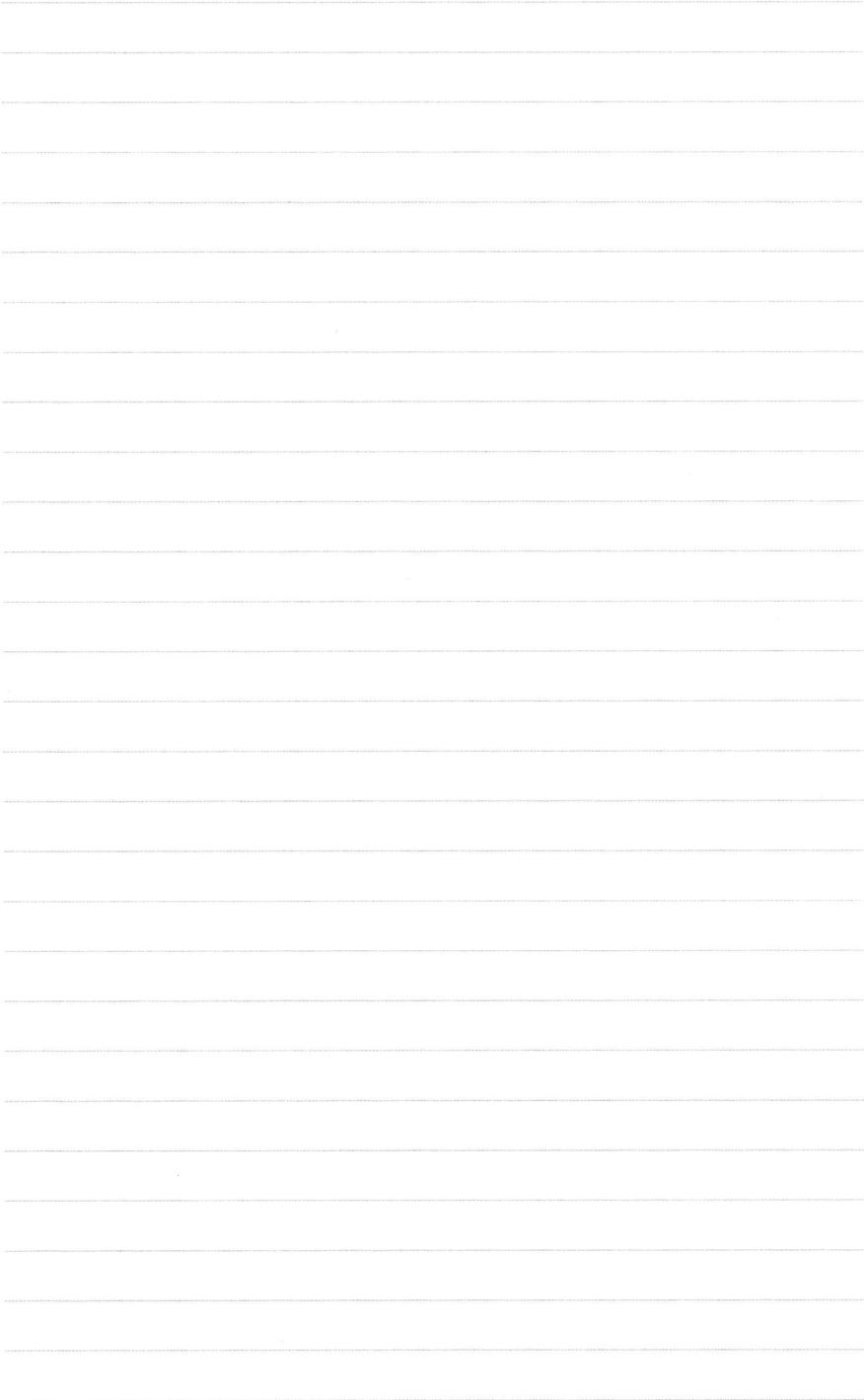

Week 39

Your body changes: Baby on the way!

If it hasn't happened yet, your baby may drop lower in your pelvis this month. Toward the end of your pregnancy, your cervix will begin to dilate. You may lose the mucous plug that's been in place at the cervical opening during your pregnancy, which can happen up to two weeks before labor begins or right before. The amniotic sac may also break or leak before labor begins. If this happens to you, follow your healthcare team's instructions. You may also have increased vaginal discharge from cervical softening and slower weight gain. And if baby has dropped, you may also feel more aches and pains in your pelvic joints.

What new body changes have arisen over the last month? Do you know what to look for when you lose your mucous plug or experience an amniotic sac leak? Have you experienced any early labor signs, such as contractions? Do you have any concerns to bring up with your healthcare team?

Did you know?

Before you were pregnant, your uterus weighed only about 2 ounces and could hold less than a half ounce. At term, it will have multiplied in weight by a factor of 20, to about 2 ½ pounds, and will have stretched to hold your baby, your placenta and almost a quart of amniotic fluid.

Stages of labor and childbirth

Every birth is different, but the sequence of events is roughly the same. Labor is divided into three natural stages. Knowing generally what to expect (and what's possible) in each stage can help you have a positive labor and birth experience.

Stage 1: The first stage of labor is the longest of the stages and is divided into three phases — early labor, active labor and transition.

Early labor begins with the start of contractions. In this phase, your cervix gradually dilates to about 6 centimeters (cm). During active labor, your contractions become stronger and progressively longer with less rest between them. Your cervix dilates more quickly, usually after about 6 cm dilation. During transitional labor, your cervix opens the remaining few centimeters, dilating all the way to 10 cm. Your contractions increase in strength and frequency with very short breaks between them.

Stage 2: Once your cervix is fully dilated and you are instructed to, you can push. It isn't unusual, especially with your first birth, to have to push for 1 to 2 hours or more before the top of your baby's head appears (crowns) at the opening of your vagina. It may still take another few minutes and a few pushes to deliver the baby.

Stage 3: The final stage of labor and childbirth is the delivery of the placenta. The placenta is the organ inside the uterus that is attached to the baby by the umbilical cord. It's the organ that has nourished your baby throughout your pregnancy.

After delivery, your healthcare team will evaluate the need for stitches or repair. More than 50% of first-time delivering parents will have stitches. Approximately 6% of people with a first delivery will have a more severe tear with increased risk for pelvic floor problems. If you have a repair, ask your care team about the severity and the repair.

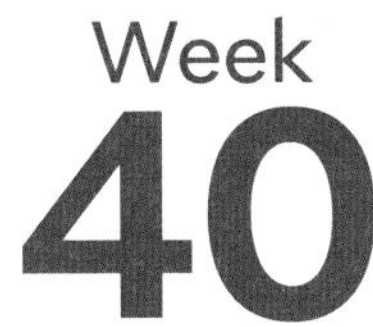

Week 40

Your baby's growth: Third trimester

Congratulations! Your due date arrives this week. And if your baby does not arrive by this week, don't fret. Most people don't deliver right on their due dates — only about 4% do.

Baby has now lost most of the lotion-like coating, called vernix, and the downy, fine hair, called lanugo, that once covered their body. However, you may still see traces of these at birth. Your baby now has enough fat laid down under the skin to hold their body temperature as long as there's a little help from you. The rest of the body has been catching up, but the head is still the largest part of your baby's body.

At 40 weeks, the average baby weighs 7 ½ to 8 pounds and measures about 20 inches long with legs fully extended. Your own baby may be smaller or larger and still be normal and healthy.

How do you feel about your baby's current size and development? Does it affect how you prepare for labor and childbirth?

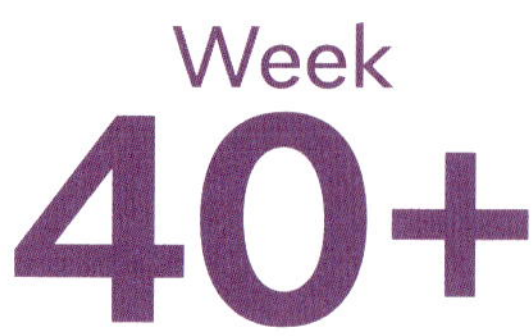

Embrace the end of pregnancy

Most people greet the end of their pregnancies with a mixture of anticipation and nervousness. Many experience a spurt of energy in the last weeks of pregnancy, often referred to as nesting. You may find yourself cleaning like mad and anxious to start any projects that you've put off.

How are you feeling overall as you reach the end of your pregnancy? Have you experienced any nesting impulses? Are there other activities you'd like to do to relax and connect with others?

Thinking about an overdue or post-term baby

If your pregnancy continues one full week past your due date, it's known as late term. Once you're two full weeks past your due date, your pregnancy is officially post-term.

To encourage labor to begin, your healthcare team may offer membrane sweeping or stripping. Or your healthcare team may recommend inducing labor.

Have you talked with your care team about options so you can help make decisions about what to try after your due date? Who can you share any worries and concerns with?

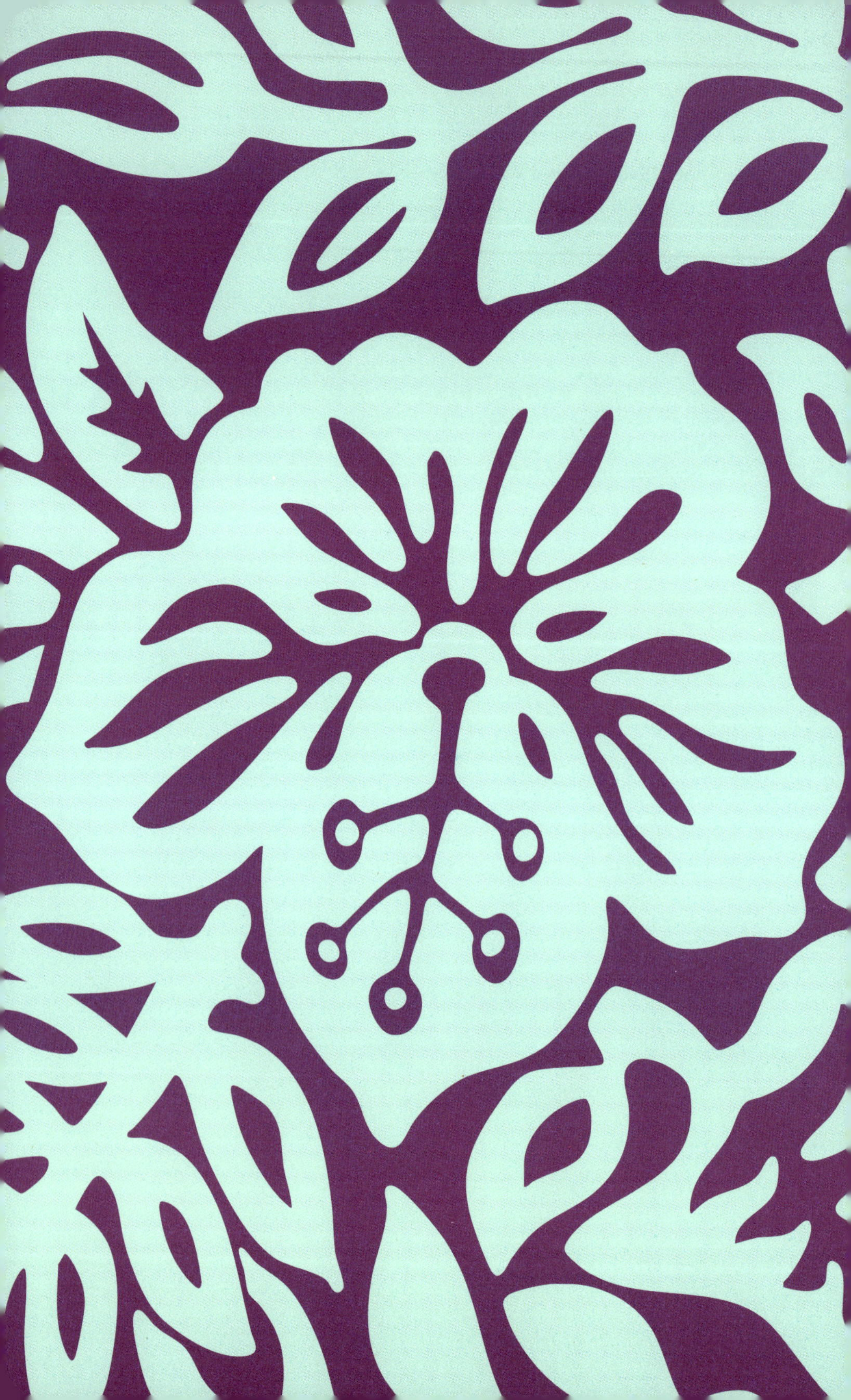

Postpartum

Your birth story

Congratulations! Your baby is finally here! Giving birth is a huge life event that can be filled with ups and downs. Take some time to write about the experience. Did you go into labor naturally, or did you have an induction or C-section? If you went into labor, when did it happen? What were the first signs? How did you spend the time before you went to the hospital?

Whether or not you went into labor naturally, what happened when you arrived at the hospital? Who was there to support you? What pain relief options did you decide to use, if any? Did you connect with any hospital staff who made the experience more positive for you? What do you remember about the progression of labor? What happened when your baby finally arrived? What was it like to meet your new baby?

Postpartum to-do list:

Here are some things to consider as you welcome your new baby into your family. You can also fill in the blank spaces with any additional items you want to consider.

- [ ] Make and go to your baby's first visit with their pediatrician or other healthcare professional
- [ ] Add your baby to your insurance plan
- [ ] Schedule your postpartum healthcare visit
- [ ] See a lactation consultant if needed
- [ ]
- [ ]
- [ ]
- [ ]
- [ ]
- [ ]
- [ ]
- [ ]
- [ ]
- [ ]
- [ ]
- [ ]
- [ ]
- [ ]

Your body changes: Postpartum

After having your baby, you may wonder if your body will ever return to normal. With a healthy lifestyle, it will! But it does take time to recover from the changes that occurred over the previous 10 months. More time than you may think! And if you're breastfeeding, that will continue to affect your body until your baby weans.

During the first days and weeks postpartum, your body will experience a great deal of changes. You may feel more tired, see stretch marks around your belly, see your skin darken in color, experience weight changes and start to deal with hair loss (but don't worry, your new look is only temporary). You might also leak urine easily, have difficulty urinating, have uterine cramping and have vaginal discharge called lochia. And you might experience bowel issues, such as constipation or fear of passing a stool, fecal incontinence and hemorrhoids. Your breasts may also go through changes such as swelling, feeling tight, increasing in size and leaking milk. You may also get sore or cracked nipples and blocked ducts. And if you dealt with any tears during labor, had any incisions made or had a C-section delivery, you may feel pain in those areas.

What body changes have you experienced since giving birth? How have you coped with these changes? Make sure to review any discharge instructions you received at the hospital, and reach out to your healthcare team if you experience any of the symptoms listed there or other concerning symptoms.

Did you know?

Expect to take at least 3 to 6 months — often longer — to get back to your pre-pregnancy shape and fitness level.

Good to know: The baby blues

Many people who recently gave birth feel depressed or anxious to some degree, a phenomenon known as the baby blues. The baby blues often include episodes of anxiety, sadness, frequent crying and exhaustion. You may find that the reality of parenthood seems difficult to cope with. The baby blues usually occur in the first two weeks after birth. Getting rest, eating a healthy diet, being as active as your body allows and expressing your feelings can help your recovery.

Have you noticed any signs or symptoms of the baby blues? What thoughts and feelings have you experienced? How can you cope with these thoughts and feelings? Who can you discuss your feelings with?

Is it more than the blues?

If signs and symptoms of the baby blues seem to be lasting longer than the first two weeks after giving birth, you may have a more severe form of mood disorder, such as postpartum depression or anxiety. For more information on the signs and symptoms of depression and anxiety, see pages 92 and 102-103.

Have your baby blues symptoms continued beyond two weeks after giving birth, or have they been severe? What symptoms are you experiencing? Who can you discuss your feelings with?

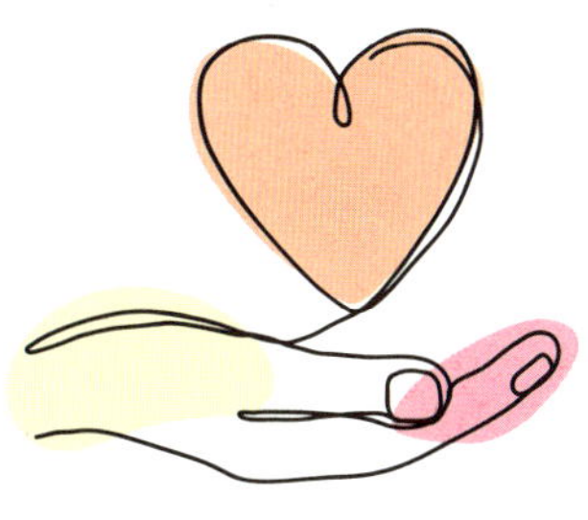

Talk with your healthcare team if you think you may have postpartum depression or anxiety. Therapy and certain medications are safe treatment options even if you're breastfeeding. Treatment can help you feel like yourself again — and be the parent your baby needs.

Appendix

THE GOOD STUFF

Here's a guide to foods that are good to eat during pregnancy, and how much of each you should aim to get each day if you're staying active.

Food category	Daily amount during pregnancy	Good choices
Grains	6 to 10 ounces	
Your body's main source of energy	1 ounce = ½ cup hot cereal or 1 cup cold cereal ½ cup cooked pasta or rice 1 slice whole-wheat bread	Whole-grain cereals, brown rice and bread, whole-wheat pasta, wild rice, quinoa, barley Tip: Look for products that list whole grains first in the ingredients list.
Vegetables	2 ½ or more cups	
Provide key vitamins and minerals and fiber	1 cup = 1 cup cooked or raw vegetables 2 cups raw leafy vegetables count as 1 cup	Lettuce, spinach, peppers, sweet potatoes, squash, peas, green beans, broccoli, carrots, corn Tips: Make a veggie pizza. Add extra vegetables to your soup, stir-fry or pasta.
Fruits	2 or more cups	
Naturally sweet and rich in nutrients and fiber	1 cup = 1 medium-sized piece of fruit 1 cup fresh, frozen or canned fruit 1 cup 100% fruit juice ½ cup dried fruit	Apples, bananas, grapes, pineapples, strawberries, blueberries, oranges, grapefruits, melons, peaches, raisins Tip: Top your cereal or yogurt with fresh fruit.

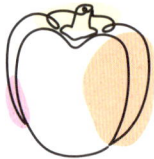

Tip: It's usually easier to eat well if you prepare more of your own food. Need recipe ideas? Check out the Healthy Recipes page at MayoClinic.org.

Based on 2020-2025 Dietary Guidelines for Americans. U.S. Department of Health and Human Services and U.S. Department of Agriculture.

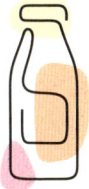

Food category	Daily amount during pregnancy	Good choices
Dairy products	3 cups	
Provide calcium, which helps build your baby's bones and teeth	1 cup = 1 cup milk 1 cup yogurt 1 ½ ounces cheese (or 2 ounces processed cheese, such as American)	Skim milk, low-fat cheese, low-fat yogurt, low-fat cottage cheese Tip: If you have trouble digesting dairy products, try soy milk fortified with calcium and vitamin D, lactose-free products and foods naturally low in lactose.
Protein foods	5 to 7 ounces	
Provide plenty of protein, which is crucial for your baby's growth 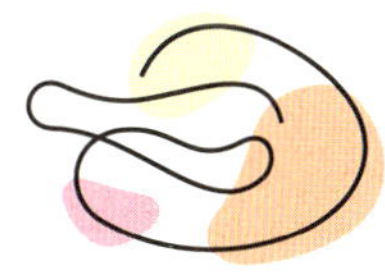	1 ounce = 1 ounce of cooked lean meat, poultry or fish 1 egg ¼ cup cooked beans ¼ cup (2 ounces) tofu 1 tablespoon peanut butter	Chicken, dried peas and beans, fish, lean beef, lean pork, peanut butter, eggs, tofu Tips: Eat whole-wheat toast with peanut butter for breakfast. Have salmon for dinner. Add chickpeas to your salad. Snack on a handful of soy nuts.
Oils	6 teaspoons	
Dense sources of energy	Oils in foods: ½ avocado = 3 teaspoons oil 1 ounce nuts = 3-4 teaspoons oil 1 tablespoon peanut butter = 2 teaspoons oil	Olive oil, nuts, seeds, avocado, salad dressing, soft margarine (trans-fat free), mayonnaise Tip: Opt for oils and fats from plant sources, which are typically low in saturated fat.
Added sugars	Eat or drink sparingly	
Extra calories that are low in nutrients		Tip: Any sugars not occurring naturally in a food (as in milk or fruit) count as added sugar, including honey and added fruit juice.

FOODS HIGH IN FOLATE (FOLIC ACID)

Food	Serving size	Folate/folic acid content
Beans	½ cup canned Great Northern beans	102 micrograms (mcg)
Spinach	½ cup cooked	89 mcg
Cereal	1 cup wheat flakes	55 mcg
Oranges	1 medium (¾ cup)	43 mcg
Asparagus	4 boiled spears (about ⅓ cup, chopped)	30 mcg
Peanuts	1 ounce dry roasted	27 mcg

FOODS HIGH IN CALCIUM

Food	Serving size	Calcium content
Yogurt	8 ounces plain, low-fat	414 milligrams (mg)
Milk	1 cup	307 mg
Juice	6 ounces orange juice fortified with calcium	262 mg
Soy milk	1 cup	237 mg
Cheese	1 ounce part-skim mozzarella	196 mg
Tahini	2 tablespoons sesame paste	128 mg
Cereal	1 cup toasted O's	110 mg
Spinach	½ cup cooked	71 mg

Based on data from USDA FoodData Central

FOODS HIGH IN PROTEIN

Food	Serving size	Protein content
Poultry	3 ounces boneless, skinless cooked chicken breast	24 grams (g)
Cottage cheese	1 cup 1% cottage cheese	25 g
Fish	3 ounces salmon	15 g
Milk	1 cup 1% milk	8 g
Peanut butter	2 tablespoons creamy	7 g
Eggs	1 large hard-boiled	6 g

FOODS HIGH IN IRON

Food	Serving size	Iron content
Cereal	1 cup wheat flakes	11 milligrams (mg)
Beans	1 cup soybeans	9 mg
Tofu	½ cup firm	3 mg
Dark chocolate	1 ounce	2 mg
Meat	3 ounces lean beef tenderloin	2 mg
Poultry	3 ounces turkey, dark meat	1 mg

Based on data from USDA FoodData Central

A MEDICATION GUIDE FOR COMMON CONDITIONS

Condition	Generally safe	Use with caution	Avoid
Allergies **Colds** **Flu**	**Nasal sprays** **Chlorpheniramine** (Chlor-Trimeton) **Acetaminophen** (Tylenol, others) **Cetirizine** (Zyrtec) **Fexofenadine** (Allegra) **Loratadine** (Claritin)	**Medications containing pseudoephedrine** (Sudafed, Claritin-D, others), especially during the first trimester **Medications containing dextromethorphan** (Robitussin, Vicks NyQuil, Vicks DayQuil, others)	**Medications containing phenylephrine** (Tylenol Allergy Multi-Symptom, others)
Constipa-tion	**Psyllium** (Metamucil) **Glycerin suppositories** (Fleet)	**Docusate** (Colace, Surfak) **Bisacodyl** (Dulcolax) **Senna** (Senokot)	**Mineral oil**
Diarrhea		**Loperamide** (Imodium A-D) for only short-term use in second and third trimesters; avoid in first trimester	**Bismuth subsalicylate** (Pepto-Bismol)
Heartburn	**Antacids** (Maalox, Tums) **Famotidine** (Pepcid) **Cimetidine** (Tagamet HB)		**Medications containing aluminum or aspirin** (Pepto-Bismol, Alka-Seltzer) Pain and fever
Pain and fever	**Acetaminophen** (Tylenol, others)	**Ibuprofen** (Advil, Motrin IB, others) only in first and second trimesters and no more than 48 hours of continuous use **Naproxen sodium** (Aleve) only in first and second trimesters and no more than 48 hours of continuous use	**Aspirin** (unless directed by your healthcare team)
Yeast infection	**Clotrimazole** (Lotrimin AF, Mycelex)	**Miconazole** (Monistat 3, Monistat 7) **Fluconazole** (Diflucan)	

HOW TO RESPOND

Your body changes so much during pregnancy that it can be hard to know which signs or symptoms need medical attention. Here's a guide to symptoms you may experience throughout your pregnancy and when you should notify your care provider. When in doubt, it's better to be safe than sorry.

Signs or symptoms	When to contact your care provider
Vaginal bleeding, spotting or discharge	
Slight spotting that goes away within a day	Within 24 hours during months 1-3; same day during months 4-7; immediately during months 8-10
Any bleeding that lasts longer than a day	Within 24 hours during months 1-3; immediately during months 4-10 or if you're Rh negative
Moderate to heavy bleeding	Immediately
Any amount of bleeding accompanied by severe pain, fever or chills	Immediately
Passing of tissue	Immediately
Greenish or yellowish vaginal discharge with odor or with vulval redness or itching	Within 24 hours
Steady or heavy discharge of watery fluid from your vagina	Immediately
Pain	
Occasional pulling or pinching sensation on one or both sides of your abdomen	Next visit
Occasional mild headaches	Next visit
A moderate, bothersome headache that doesn't go away	Within 24 hours
A severe or persistent headache, especially with dizziness, faintness, nausea or vomiting, or visual disturbances	Immediately
Moderate to severe pelvic pain	Immediately
Any degree of pelvic pain that doesn't subside within 4 hours	Within 24 hours
Pain with fever or bleeding	Immediately
Leg pain with redness and swelling	Immediately
Uterine contractions, less than six each hour for 2 or more hours	Next visit
Uterine contractions, more than six each hour for 2 or more hours	Immediately

Signs or symptoms	When to contact your care provider
Vomiting	
Occasional or once daily	Next visit
More than three times daily with inability to eat or drink	Within 24 hours
Accompanied by pain or fever	Immediately
Other	
Fever lower than 102°F	Within 24 hours if fever persists
Fever of 102°F or higher	Immediately
Painful urination	Same day
Inability to urinate	Same day
Mild constipation	Next visit
Severe constipation, no bowel movement for 3 days	Same day
Consistently low mood, loss of pleasure	Next visit
Low mood, loss of pleasure, and thoughts of harming yourself or others	Immediately
Cravings for nonfood substances such as clay or dirt	Next visit
Sudden swelling of hands, face or feet	Same day
Sudden weight gain	Same day
Fainting or visual disturbances (blurring)	Immediately
Fatigue, weakness, shortness of breath, heart palpitations or lightheadedness	Next visit if occurring occasionally; same day if persistent
Severe shortness of breath	Immediately
Severe itching	Same day

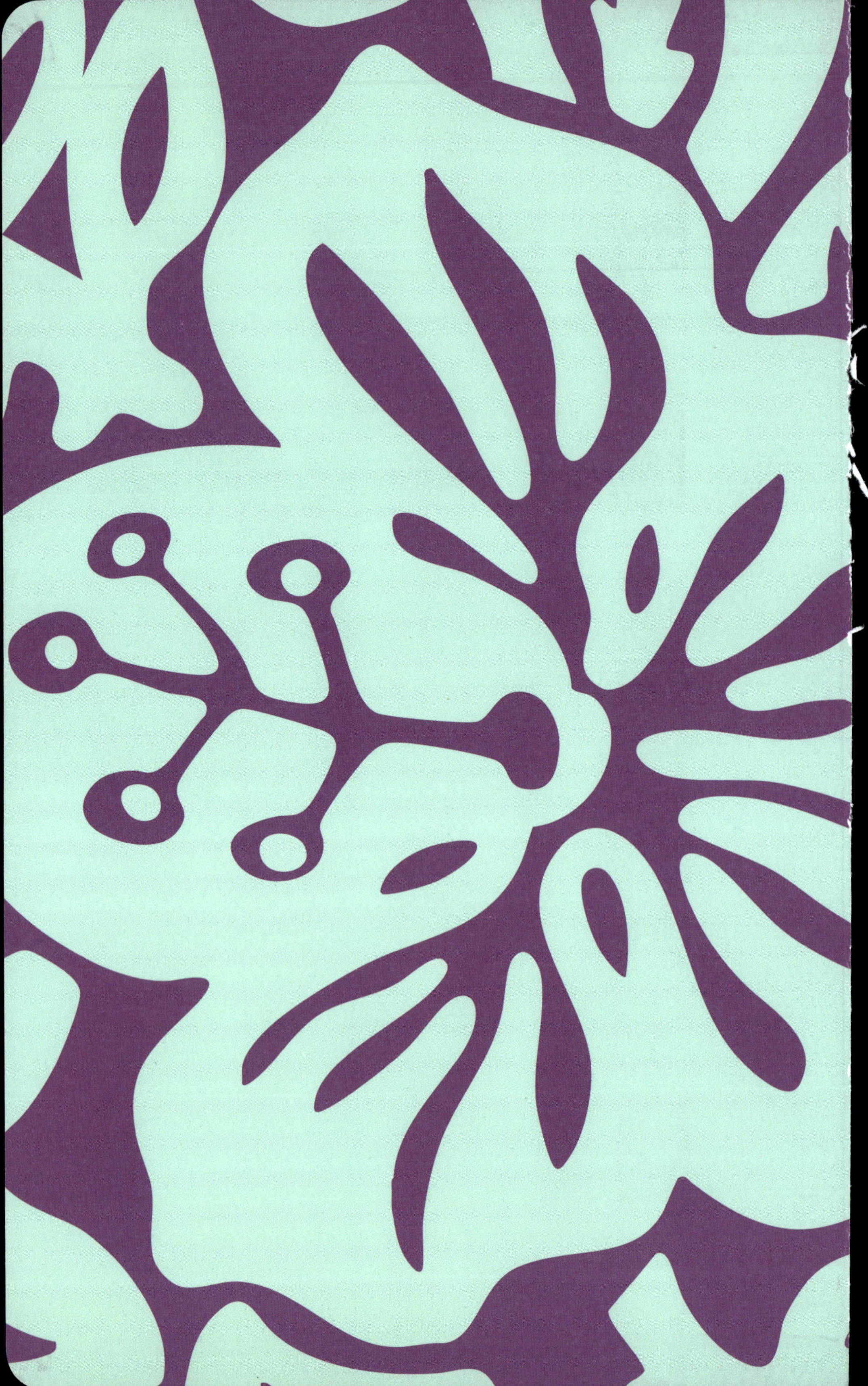